**Zaki Boudiaf**

# Colorectal cancer with synchronous liver metastases

**Zaki Boudiaf**

# Colorectal cancer with synchronous liver metastases

## Place of laparoscopic surgery

**ScienciaScripts**

**Imprint**



Cover image: www.ingimage.com

This book is a translation from the original published under ISBN 978-620-6-72405-6.

Publisher:
Sciencia Scripts
is a trademark of
Dodo Books Indian Ocean Ltd. and OmniScriptum S.R.L publishing group

120 High Road, East Finchley, London, N2 9ED, United Kingdom
Str. Armeneasca 28/1, office 1, Chisinau MD-2012, Republic of Moldova, Europe
Printed at: see last page
**ISBN: 978-620-8-26855-8**

# Colorectal cancer with synchronous liver metastases.

## Place of laparoscopic surgery

Zaki Boudiaf MD, PhD

Surgical Oncology "A" Department

Center Pierre et Marie Curie, Algiers Algeria

Contents

# I. Introduction - Issues :

## A. Epidemiology :

Colorectal cancer (CRC) is the world's third most common cancer in terms of incidence, after lung and breast cancer. In 2018, its incidence was estimated at 1.8 million new cases, or 10.2% of all cancer cases. (1) (Fig.1).

In the same year, it was responsible for the deaths of 88,1000 people worldwide (9.2%), making it the second leading cause of cancer deaths after lung cancer. (1) (Fig.2).

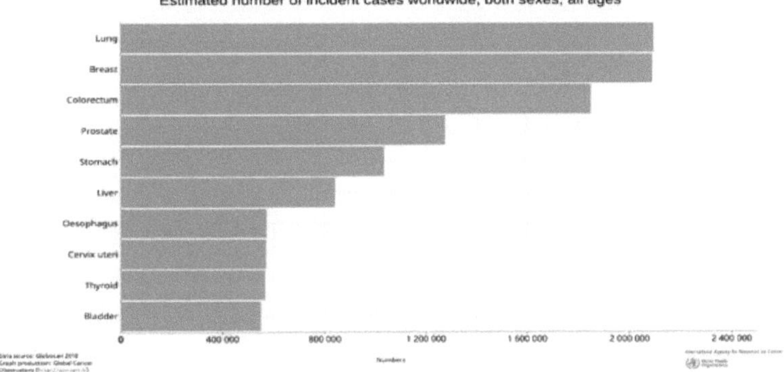


**Figure 1** Incidence by type of cancer worldwide (1).

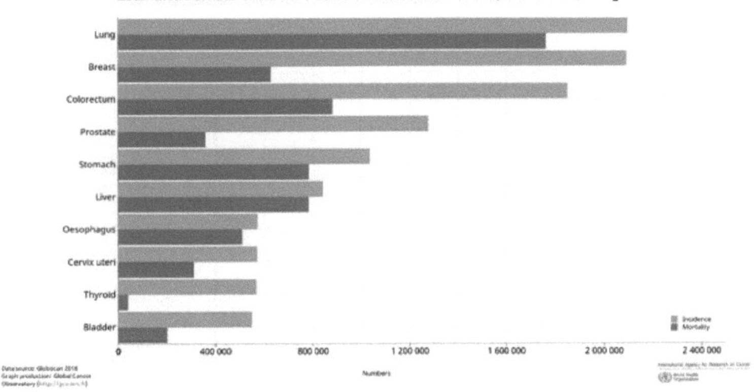


**Figure 2** Incidence and mortality by type of cancer worldwide (1).

By gender, lung cancer is the most frequently diagnosed cancer and the leading cause of cancer death in men, followed by prostate and colorectal cancer for incidence, and liver and stomach cancer for mortality. In women, breast cancer is the most frequently diagnosed cancer and the leading cause of cancer death, followed by colorectal cancer and lung cancer for incidence, and vice versa for mortality. (1) (Fig.3, Fig.4).

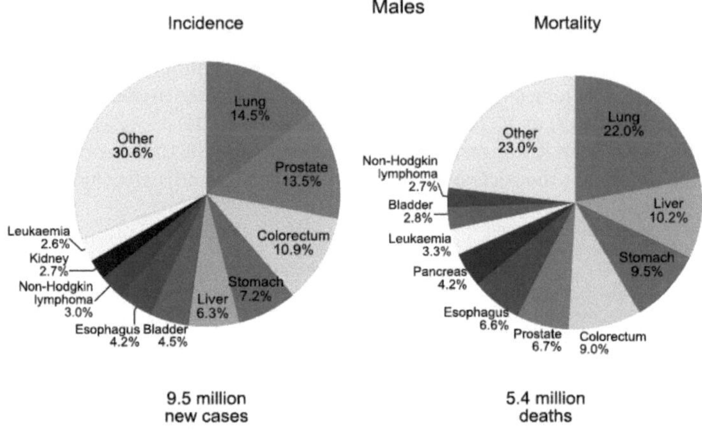


**Figure 3** Incidence and mortality by type of cancer in men worldwide (1).

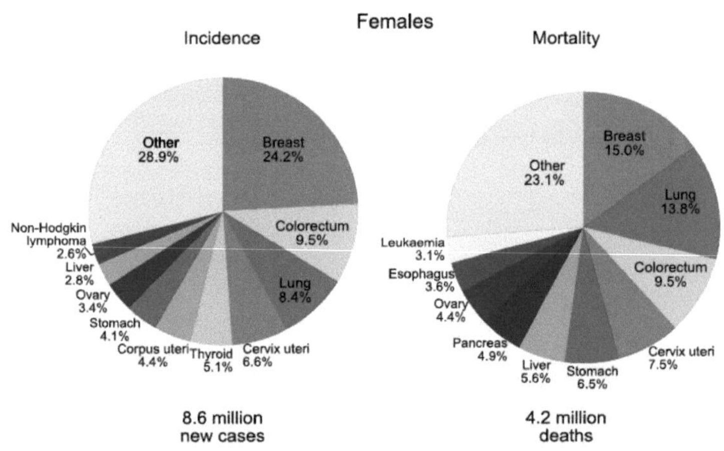


**Figure 4** Incidence and mortality by type of cancer in women worldwide (1).

The highest colorectal cancer incidence rates have been reported in Western countries, with an age-standardized rate ≥ 26.8 per 100,000 in 2018 (2) (Fig.5).

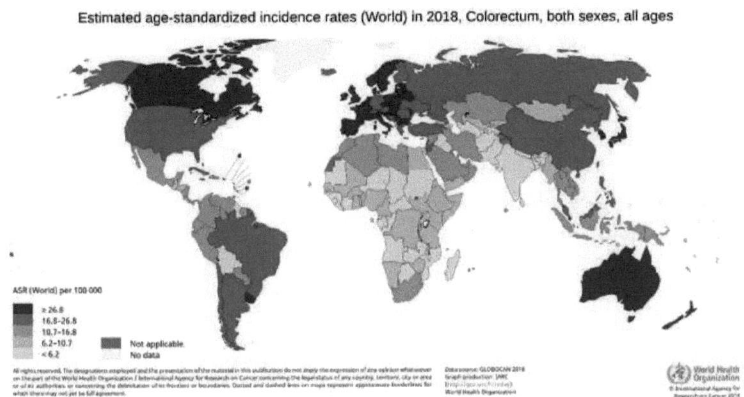


**Figure 5** Age-standardized incidence of colorectal cancer by country in 2018 (2).

In Algeria, the age-standardized incidence rate was 13.9 per 100,000 in 2018. As a result, Algeria is considered a medium-incidence country. (3) (Fig.6). Nevertheless, colorectal cancer is the $1^{er}$ digestive cancer, its uninterrupted progression since the mid-2000s now placing it in second place in both men and women (4) (Fig.7, Fig.8). It is also considered the second leading cause of cancer death in Algeria for both sexes (3) (Fig.7, Fig.8).

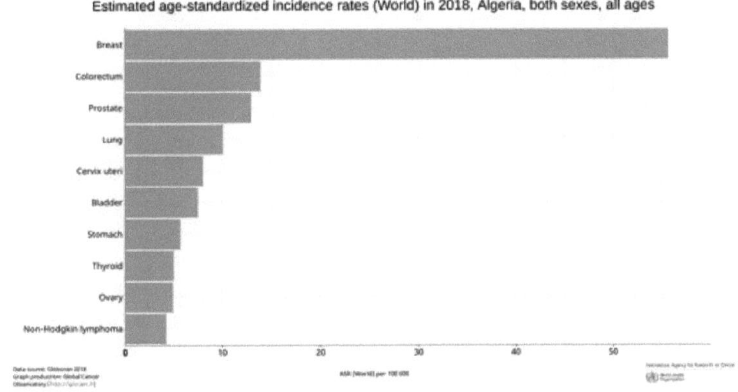


**Figure 6** Age-standardized incidence rate in Algeria in 2018 (3).

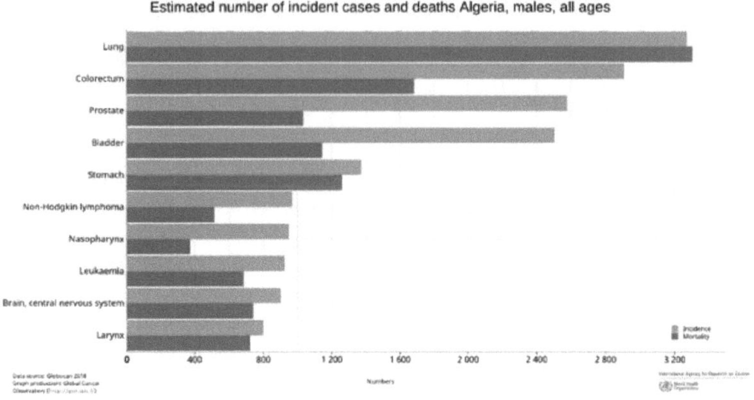


**Figure 7** Incidence and mortality of colorectal cancer in men in Algeria in 2018. (3).

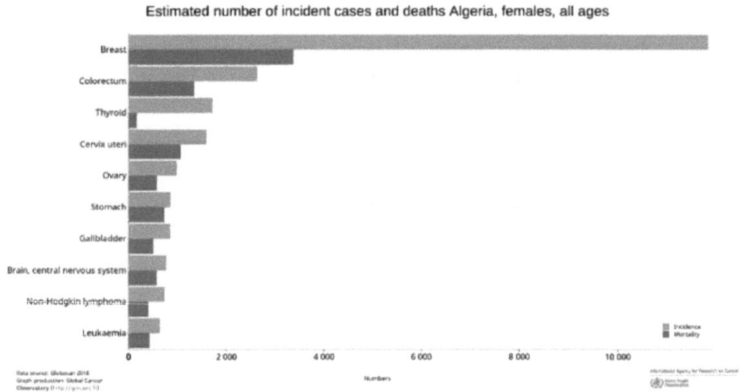


**Figure 8** Incidence and mortality of colorectal cancer in women in Algeria in 2018. (3).

In Algiers, according to tumor registry data updated in 2017 (5)colorectal cancer ranks first in men and second after breast cancer in women, with an increasing trend in incidence over the last decade in both sexes (5) (Fig.09,Fig.10,Fig.11,Fig.12).

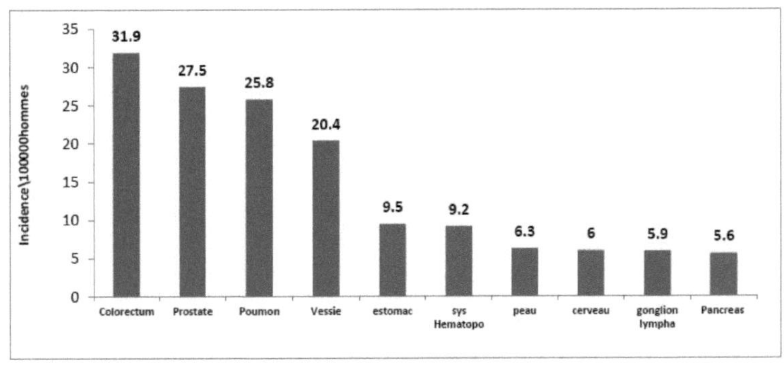


**Figure 9** Most frequent cancer sites in men in Algiers in 2017 (5).

| | 2008 | 2009 | 2010 | 2011 | 2012 | 2013 | 2014 | 2015 | 2016 | 2017 |
|---|---|---|---|---|---|---|---|---|---|---|
| Colon rectum | 12.5 | 20.36 | 15.7 | 16.8 | 19.4 | 23.4 | 23.1 | 24.2 | 25.2 | 31.9 |

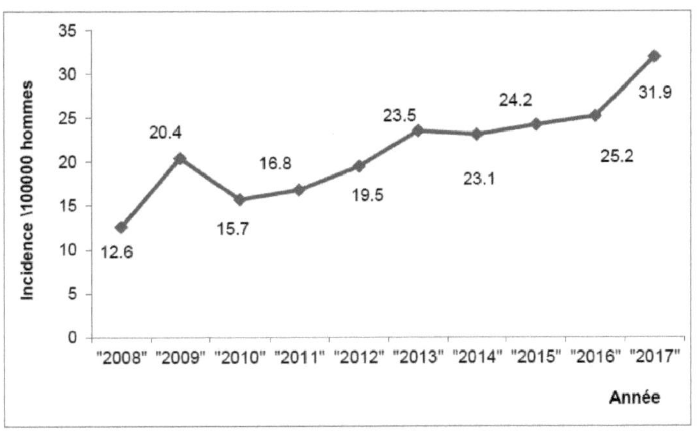


**Figure 10** Colorectal cancer trends in men in Algiers 2008 - 2017 (5).

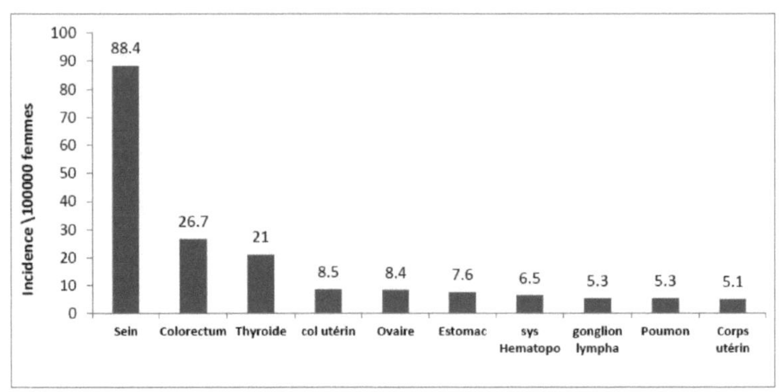


**Figure 11** Most frequent cancer sites in women in Algiers in 2017 (5).

| | 2008 | 2009 | 2010 | 2011 | 2012 | 2013 | 2014 | 2015 | 2016 | 2017 |
|---|---|---|---|---|---|---|---|---|---|---|
| Colon rectum | 11.7 | 13.9 | 16.7 | 16.8 | 18.3 | 19 | 21.6 | 22.7 | 21,7 | 26.7 |

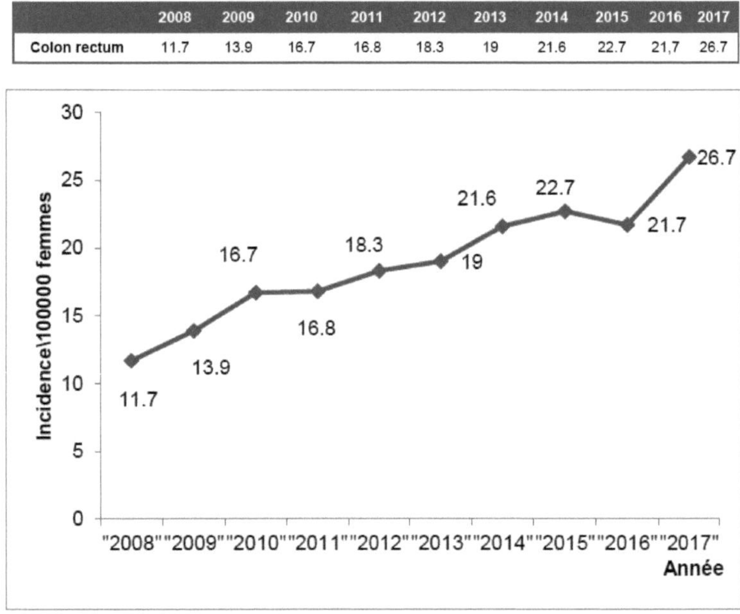


**Figure 12** Colorectal cancer trends in women in Algiers 2008 - 2017 (5).

## B. Evolution of ideas and issues :

Colorectal cancer is the leading digestive cancer in Algeria (4)it is also considered the second leading cause of cancer deaths for both sexes (3).

Survival is determined by tumour stage, with a 5-year survival rate of 90.3% for stage I and only 12.5% for stage IV. (6).
Stage IV is the metastatic stage of the disease, and the liver is the most frequent site of CRC metastases.
During the course of the disease, 40-60% of patients will develop liver metastases, which are synchronous in 10-25% of cases. (7).
If left untreated, the prognosis is poor (median survival 9-12 months). Excisional surgery is the only potentially curative treatment, with 5-year survival ranging from 35% to 58%. Mortality and morbidity after surgery are respectively less than 5% and 25%, but excisional surgery is only possible in 15 to 30% of metastatic patients. (7).
The clinical presentation of patients with synchronous liver metastases is highly variable, depending on the site (colon or rectum), the stage of the primary tumor and the extent of metastatic disease. Consequently, management differs from one presentation to the next.
The therapeutic strategy for patients with synchronous liver metastases from colorectal cancer (MHSCCR) is still under debate.
To date, the optimal timing for surgical resection of synchronous liver metastases is not well defined and remains controversial (8).
The classic approach is a sequential one, involving initial resection of the primary colorectal tumor followed by liver resection around 2-3 months later (9)This strategy makes it possible to select patients for secondary liver resection, excluding those with progressing metastatic disease, and therefore improves oncological outcomes.
This tumor progression during chemotherapy has traditionally been regarded as a biological selection process for patients prior to hepatectomy, and is now increasingly regarded as a loss of chance of cure (more than 30% of cases). (10).
Recent advances in chemotherapy, notably the introduction of targeted therapies, and in liver surgery, with volume-conserving resections and re-hepatectomies, preoperative manipulation of liver volume and patient optimization, have enabled surgeons to adopt new approaches to the conventional treatment of synchronous liver metastases from colorectal cancer.
With this in mind, in 2006 G.Mentha described the reverse or liver-first approach (11)which is also a sequential approach, but where resection of liver metastases precedes that of the primary focus.
Quoted by Polignano (10)T.Ishizawa observed that the interval to the second operation was significantly longer when colon resection was performed first (130 vs. 49 days, $p < 0.01$).
It was also observed that liver metastasis growth was accelerated by resecting the primary tumor due to changes in tumor homeostasis and the elimination of angiogenesis-inhibiting factors (12).
Moreover, liver metastases are considered to be the main determinant of patient prognosis, and it is the opinion of many authors that they should be treated first and as early as possible, particularly if the primary tumor is asymptomatic.
On the other hand, other authors have reported a simultaneous approach (colorectal and liver resection are combined), which was beneficial in terms of

post-operative results with a shorter hospital stay. Indeed, several studies had concluded that this strategy was safe and effective in terms of both oncology and post-operative outcomes, with mortality and morbidity rates comparable with those of the sequential approach, and a potential reduction in total hospital stay (13).
Several reports, including J.Chen's meta-analysis (14)have shown the benefit of simultaneous open resection of the primary tumor and synchronous colorectal liver metastases, compared with a sequential approach.
Synchronous resections have the advantage of requiring only a single procedure to treat both tumour sites, a shorter hospital stay and shorter operating time compared to the combined results of sequential resections. This single procedure also reduces psychological stress for patients, who won't have to wait for a second procedure with the tumor in place.
Simultaneous liver and colorectal resection for cancer with synchronous metastases was long practised, but was often associated with a perceived increased risk of complications and mortality until the late 1990s (15).
High morbidity and mortality rates have been attributed to the association of clean surgery (liver) with surgery at risk of contamination (colorectal). In addition, disruption of liver function after resection could leave the patient vulnerable to infection and increase the risk of anastomotic fistula. Also, clamping the hepatic pedicle causes portal hypertension, which may impair colonic anastomosis through intestinal edema, increasing the risk of fistula (16).
These risks remain hypothetical because numerous recent studies suggest that colorectal and liver resections are possible and can be performed with acceptable morbidity and without compromising long-term survival. (17-19). The meta-analysis by J.Chen (14) comparing simultaneous versus sequential resection of synchronous liver metastases confirmed these results, with the simultaneous approach having the advantage (significant difference) of shorter operative time, less blood loss, shorter hospital stay and reduced morbidity.
Survival at 3 years was also in favor of simultaneous resections, in the comparative study of 228 patients at the Paul Brousse hepatobiliary center, published in 2010 by De Haas (20).
Major hepatectomies can also be combined with colorectal resections, but caution is advised when such an approach is attempted due to reports of increased morbidity. Reddy (21) in a multi-institutional analysis showed that, compared with a sequential approach, synchronous resection resulted in shorter hospitalization and lower morbidity for minor hepatectomies, but morbidity was higher when major hepatectomies were performed (36.1 vs. 17.6%).
Simultaneous surgery therefore appears to be of interest for patients who do not require major liver resection, and who have an uncomplicated primary colorectal tumor.
Focusing on the technical aspects, the main problem with combined surgery is the need for an adequate abdominal approach, particularly for left colon and rectal cancer, which require a long midline abdominal incision with frequent subcostal splitting for liver surgery, considered a debilitating approach not devoid of early

or distant morbidity and which could lead the surgeon to defer treatment of one of the two tumor sites.
To overcome this difficulty of adequate and optimal exposure, a laparoscopic approach to one or both tumor sites could facilitate this simultaneous approach.
Laparoscopic surgery, designed to reduce surgical stress and the pain associated with large incisions, tends to improve short-term results and give similar long-term results.
The introduction and development of laparoscopic techniques have greatly contributed to the improvement of short-term post-surgery outcomes over the past two decades. Laparoscopic colorectal resection has been shown to be safe and effective in several large randomized trials (22,23) and has been accepted as an alternative to the conventional route.
Although laparoscopic liver resection was introduced at the same time as colorectal resection (the first laparoscopic liver resection was reported in 1992 by M.Gagner (24)), the wide diffusion of this procedure was hampered by its technical difficulties and by oncological concerns about transsection of a solid organ. More recently, with technological evolution and improved surgical experience, laparoscopy for liver resection has become an established technique (25).
Thus, hepatobiliary surgeons from selected specialized centers reported that laparoscopic liver resection was feasible and safe, not only for benign pathologies, but also for hepatocellular carcinomas or colorectal liver metastases (26).
Concerns about potential uncontrollable bleeding, gas embolism, oncological inadequacy of the resection and loss of tactile sense (which can help identify intraparenchymal lesions) have slowed the development of laparoscopic liver resection techniques.
Nevertheless, as experience accumulated, hepatobiliary surgeons in selected specialized centers began reporting laparoscopic resections. Studies of thousands of cases of laparoscopic liver resection concluded that laparoscopy was associated with less morbidity, less pain, faster recovery, shorter hospital stay than open procedures, without compromising oncologic clearance (25,26).
As a result, and in order to avoid the need for an invasive approach, and to be able to operate under good exposure conditions on both surgical sites (colorectal and hepatic), the laparoscopic approach to one or both surgical sites seems attractive, and would reduce the parietal trauma that is one of the major drawbacks of the combined laparotomy approach. The potential advantages of this approach are the possibility of performing a radical operation with small incisions, improved rehabilitation and reduced costs.
Reduced hospital stays and more rapid referral to adjuvant treatment are key advantages of the laparoscopic approach over conventional surgery. In addition, by reducing postoperative adhesions, laparoscopy enables easier access in the event of re-hepatectomy for recurrence.
Only small series of simultaneous laparoscopic colorectal and liver resections have been published to date, most using a hybrid technique combining a laparoscopic approach to the primary colorectal tumor and a laparotomy approach to the liver metastasis, or a hand-assisted technique.

The totally laparoscopic approach remains the preserve of hepatic metastases in the anteroinferior segments (II-III-IV-V-VI), which are more accessible and require minor hepatic resections < 3 segments (27). Nevertheless, posterior segment resections and major laparoscopic resections have been reported in the literature, usually in the form of case reports or limited series.

The first cases of simultaneous laparoscopic resection of a colorectal tumor and its liver metastasis were reported in 2006 .

T.M Geiger (28) reported a case entitled "Laparoscopic resection of colon cancer and synchronous liver metastasis" in a 60-year-old patient with sigmoid adenocarcinoma and single left lobe metastasis. A hepatic resection (hand-assisted left lobectomy) followed by a laparoscopic sigmoid resection had been performed with simple postoperative follow-up and good carcinological quality.

K.L Leung (29) published another case report in the same journal, entitled "Simultaneous laparoscopic resection of rectal cancer and liver metastasis". This time, it concerned a totally laparoscopic resection combining an anterior resection for cancer of the upper rectum followed by a left lobectomy for a double metastatic localization in a 53-year-old patient, with a simple postoperative course and R0 quality resection of both tumour sites.

Since then, a host of publications have been published on this new approach.

F.Bretagnol (18) in 2008 had already reported in his preliminary experience the benefit of laparoscopic resection of rectal cancer in patients undergoing simultaneous laparotomy surgery for synchronous liver metastases, in a short series of ten patients. A larger series of 51 patients from the same Beaujon Hospital team was published in 2013 by C.Hatwell (30) under the title "Laparoscopic resection of colorectal cancer facilitates simultaneous surgery of synchronous liver metastases", the author concluded that laparoscopic colorectal resection combined with open, or laparoscopic, liver resection for synchronous liver metastases was feasible and safe, and did not compromise postoperative outcome. Moreover, laparoscopy appeared to facilitate the surgical approach for combined liver resection.

In the same vein, JW.Huh (31) in 2011 reviewed 40 consecutive patients who had undergone simultaneous R0 resection for synchronous liver metastases of colorectal cancers, among whom 20 patients had undergone simultaneous laparoscopic colorectal resection, matched with 20 patients operated on via the conventional route. No significant difference in postoperative complications was observed between the two groups. The 3-year overall survival rate in the laparoscopic group was not significantly different from that in the laparotomy group (52.8 vs. 61.0%, $p$ = 0.713). The author concluded that laparoscopic colorectal resection, combined with resection of liver metastases, had a similar outcome to the open approach but offered some short-term advantages.

In 2015 F.Ratti (32) published a comparative study between two groups of patients operated on for metastatic colorectal cancer; a first group of 69 patients who had laparoscopic colorectal resection combined with laparotomy liver resection, to a second group of 37 patients who had simultaneous laparotomy colorectal and liver resection. A retrospective comparative analysis of these two groups concluded that laparoscopic resection of colorectal cancer in patients undergoing simultaneous laparotomy for liver metastases was associated with reduced blood loss, morbidity and postoperative hospital stay, without affecting oncological radicality. The post-operative course was mainly determined by the type of approach to colorectal surgery, rather than the extent of liver resection.

K.U Jung (33) in 2014 in a retrospective study, with matched-case analysis of prospectively collected data, had compared 24 patients who had simultaneous laparoscopic colorectal and liver resection (laparoscopy group), with 24 patients who had simultaneous laparotomy resection (laparotomy group N = 24 of 232).

His analysis had concluded that a totally laparoscopic approach could offer short-term advantages with better postoperative rehabilitation despite a longer procedure. This approach could be considered a reasonable option in simultaneous colorectal and liver resections.

In a systematic review by R.M. Lupinacci (34) and published in 2014, on simultaneous laparoscopic resections of primary colorectal cancer and associated liver metastases, and which aimed to identify all the data in the literature concerning the feasibility and short-term results of this combined laparoscopic approach (liver resection was considered if ≥ 2 resected segments).

Its database was drawn from case reports, case series and case-control studies. Thirty-nine cases of simultaneous minimally invasive resection were reported in fourteen publications included in this systematic review. In his commentary he wrote "the simultaneous laparoscopic approach is the first choice for selected cases, but there are no large series published in the literature. The most likely reason is that these procedures would require a surgeon with experience in both laparoscopic colorectal and liver surgery, or cooperation between two different teams".

His conclusion was that, despite the lack of high-quality evidence, laparoscopy in this combined approach appeared to be feasible and safe, even for major hepatectomies. Good patient selection and refined surgical technique were the keys to successful simultaneous resection.

The most important Report published to date on laparoscopic synchronous resection of CRC and liver metastases, is an international multicenter study involving 142 patients (France, USA, Italy and South Korea) published in World journal of surgery and reported by S.Ferretti in 2015 (35).

The conversion rate was 4.9%, overall morbidity 31.0% and mortality 2.1%. Overall survival at 1, 3 and 5 years was 98.8 - 82.1 and 71.9% respectively.

By multivariate analysis, ASA score ≥3 [OR 13.6 (1.8-99.6); $p = 0.01$] and operative time [OR 1.008 (1.001-1.016); $p = 0.03$] were two independent predictors of postoperative morbidity.

The study concluded that in experienced centers, the simultaneous laparoscopic approach was technically feasible, safe and associated with good oncological outcomes.

This international multicenter series of 142 patients was the subject of another publication the same year by H.Tranchart (36) in "Surgical Endoscopy", the aim of which was to compare short- and long-term results for matched patients having undergone combined resections (laparoscopy vs. laparotomy) using a propensity

score. This international multicenter database of 142 patients was compared with a database of 241 patients treated by laparotomy during the same period.
After matching, 89 patients were compared in each group.
There was no difference in overall operative time, blood loss or transfusion rate between the two groups. Conversion was necessary in 7% of cases in the laparoscopic group. Morbidity rates were similar in both groups ($p = 1.0$).
Overall survival at 3 years in the laparoscopy and laparotomy groups was 78% and 65% respectively ($p = 0.17$).
More recently in 2016, another review of the literature was published by S.Garritano (37)which aimed to analyze the perioperative and oncological outcomes of simultaneous minimally invasive resection of colorectal cancer and synchronous liver metastases. Twenty clinical reports were included in this review, encompassing 150 patients. The approach was laparoscopic in 139 patients (92.7%) and robotic in 11 patients (7.3%). The primary tumor was rectal in 52.7% of cases. Combined liver surgery was a minor hepatic resection in 89% of cases. One patient (0.7%) required conversion to open surgery. The overall morbidity and mortality rates were 18% and 1.3% respectively. The most frequent complication was anastomotic fistula (3.3%).
Data on oncological outcomes were too heterogeneous to provide definitive results.
He concluded that, although no prospective randomized trials were available, laparoscopic simultaneous resection appeared to offer advantages over conventional surgery in terms of short-term postoperative results. On the other hand, more studies were needed to define the oncological values of combined minimally invasive treatment.
In 2019 Mr. J. van der Poel (38) published for the first time a multicenter comparative study using a propensity score comparing 61 patients with MHSCCR (operated on by combined laparoscopic approach), with 61 patients with CRC resected laparoscopically.
Simultaneous laparoscopic surgery with minor hepatectomy could be performed safely without increasing the risk of postoperative morbidity compared with laparoscopic colorectal resection alone.
In more complex liver optimization strategies, in the management of bilobar hepatic metastases involving two-stage hepatectomy, the laparoscopic approach during the first operative stage, combining resection of the primary tumor and a hepatic procedure of resection or radiofrequency thermoablation or portal ligation, would facilitate the second operative stage, which often requires a major hepatectomy. These advantages have been reported by P. Pessaux (39) in a letter to the editor commenting on the article by F.Bretagnol (18).
To date, and through a review of international publications on the subject, the data collected are limited to observational studies and literature reviews, which may present biases, given the multifactorial technical complexity of laparoscopy, patient selection and stage of disease. Current data in the literature do not allow definitive conclusions to be drawn on the place of laparoscopy in the overall therapeutic strategy for the management of colorectal cancers with synchronous liver metastases.

Moreover, no study on this subject has yet been published or initiated in Algeria. With this in mind, we aim to evaluate this minimally invasive approach from the standpoint of technical feasibility and carcinological safety, and consequently define from a prospective study of a group of patients with MHSCCR the place of minimally invasive surgery in the combined strategy of therapeutic management of these patients.

This group of patients will be compared, as in the study by M. J. van der Poel, with a group of patients undergoing laparoscopic colorectal cancer surgery.

# II. Natural history /oncogenesis - dissemination :

## A. Natural history of cancer:

The natural history of cancer can be divided schematically into several stages: the cancerous transformation of a cell; the clonal expansion of the cancer cell; the growth of the tumor mass, followed by the dissemination of cancer cells away from the initial tumor site, and the formation of secondary tumor sites (metastases).

This tumor progression is linked to the genetic instability of cancer cells. Spontaneous genetic changes occur progressively, with the appearance of variants of the initial clone, resulting in tumor heterogeneity. These variant clones will have heterogeneous proliferative, invasive, antigenic and metastatic behaviours, or unequal sensitivity to chemotherapy (40).

### 1. Local phase of cancer: invasion

#### *a) Diagnostic importance, notion of microinvasive carcinoma :*

From the epithelium, carcinoma cells erode the basement membrane and invade the superficial part of the underlying chorion. At this stage, the carcinoma is termed "microinvasive". These superficial invasive cancers generally have a better prognosis than more advanced cancers of the same type.

#### *b) Local invasion:*

The tumor progressively extends into the organ in which it originated, invading its various constituents one by one (e.g. submucosa, then colonic muscularis...). Normal tissue is gradually replaced by tumor formation. In a solid organ (liver, kidney), it forms a single, rounded mass.

In a hollow organ such as the digestive tract, it invades the different planes of the wall more or less rapidly and successively.

Invasive cancer destroys normal tissues, preferentially using pathways of least resistance to spread: loose connective spaces, peri-nervous spaces, lymphatic and blood capillaries, venous walls. Cancer cells can disperse in isolation in connective tissue, far removed from the main tumour mass, and cause local recurrence.

By contiguity, the tumor then invades neighboring organs and adjacent structures: this is regional extension.

### 2. General cancer phase: metastasis

#### *a) Definitions :*

Tumor progression depends on proliferative and metastasizing capacity.

After a local phase, metastasis (from the Greek metastasis: displacement) is the most serious aspect of cancer.

Metastases are secondary cancerous foci that develop at a distance from the primary tumor, and whose growth is autonomous, independent of that of the primary tumor.

A very small proportion of circulating tumor cells are capable of forming a metastasis: less than one in 10,000 tumor cells that leave the primary tumor escape the body's defense system and form a new tumor.

Due to their genetic and phenotypic heterogeneity, the various cancer cells of a single tumor have varying metastatic capacities: the natural history of a cancer involves a positive selection of cellular sub-clones with metastasizing capacity.

### *b) Different stages of metastatic spread*

Whether by blood or lymphatic route, cancer cells leaving the initial tumor site must pass through successive stages, each of which represents an obstacle that only a small number of cancer cells that have succeeded in adapting to a new environment will be able to overcome. (41).

These different stages are: cell detachment and invasion of the extra-cellular matrix; intravasation (passage into the circulation); survival in the circulation; extravasation; survival and proliferation in a foreign site.

### *c) Different migration routes*

Migration of tumour cells away from the primary site can take place via several routes, the relative importance of which depends very much on the type of tumour. The main routes are lymphatic and blood-borne, but there may also be diffusion via the body's natural cavities (peritoneal serosa, etc.).

#### (1) Lymphatic extension

This is the most common route of dissemination for carcinomas, but can also occur in sarcomas.

Lymph node metastasis is based on normal lymph node drainage in the affected region.

The first lymph node in lymphatic drainage is called the sentinel node.

As the lymphatic invasion progresses, cancer cells are released into the general circulation via the thoracic duct. A frequent intermediate stage is the presence of a left supra-clavicular lymph node (Troisier lymph node), the last relay before the general circulation, and thus a sign that the cancerous process is about to spread throughout the body.

#### (2) Hematogenous extension

Cancer cells, either after passing through the lymphatic pathway or directly by breaking through the blood vessel wall, penetrate the small blood vessels and are carried by the circulation to the organs that filter the largest volume of blood.

This is made all the easier by the thin walls of the stromal vessels.

#### (3) Direct swarming through a natural cavity:

It can occur when a malignant tumor extends into this cavity, such as the pleural or peritoneal cavities, meningeal spaces, urinary tracts, bile ducts or a joint cavity. Examples: peritoneal extension of ovarian carcinoma, ovarian extension of gastric adenocarcinoma (Krükenberg tumor).

This swarming can also occur when the tumor ruptures in a cavity.

## B. Carcinogenesis of colorectal cancer:

Colorectal carcinogenesis is a complex process essentially linked to successive genetic alterations. The accumulation of these genetic anomalies leads to the appearance of an aberrant crypt, then an adenoma, then colorectal cancer.

### 1. Main mechanisms of colorectal carcinogenesis :

Cancer is a multi-stage genetic disease, corresponding to the acquisition of characteristic properties such as autonomous growth, escape from apoptosis, insensitivity to antiproliferative signals, increased angiogenesis, unlimited replication potential, metastatic invasion and escape from immunosurveillance.

Colorectal carcinogenesis is mainly linked to 3 major mechanisms: chromosomal instability (75% of CRCs), microsatellite instability (15% of CRCs) and CpG island hypermethylation (25% of CRCs), which are not mutually exclusive.

Most CRCs are of sporadic origin (70%), but in a minority of cases, germline genetic alterations are at the origin of the carcinogenesis process. The two best-defined familial forms are Lynch syndrome or HNPCC (hereditary non polyposis colorectal cancer) and familial adenomatous polyposis. A proportion of CRCs (20-30%) are thought to have a hereditary component linked to alleles with low penetrance or oligogenic determinism. Chronic inflammation and certain environmental factors, notably nutritional, promote colorectal carcinogenesis. (42). Thus, the different pathways of colorectal carcinogenesis are complex and not mutually exclusive (43) (Fig.13).

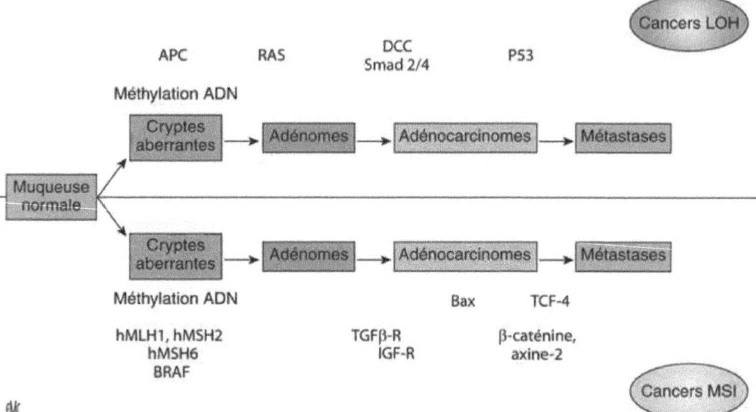


**Figure 13** Two mechanisms of colonic carcinogenesis: loss of heterozygosity and microsatellite instability (42).

### 2. Precancerous colorectal lesions :

In the majority of cases, transformation of the colonic epithelium follows the adenoma-dysplasia-cancer filiation. RCCs develop from precancerous lesions, **the** aberrant **crypt** (44) which represents the first identifiable lesion corresponding to an abnormality in the opening of crypts in the form of an enlarged opening associated with epithelial hyperplasia, evolving towards adenoma. **Adenomas** are

associated with lesions of varying degrees of dysplasia, progressing to **intramucosal adenocarcinoma** and then to **invasive tumours**.
In aberrant crypts, it is possible to identify certain molecular abnormalities such as *KRAS* (*kirsten rat sarcoma viral oncogene homolog*) or *APC* mutation, microsatellite instability or hypermethylation of CpG islets, suggesting that these are early events in carcinogenesis (45) (Fig. 14).

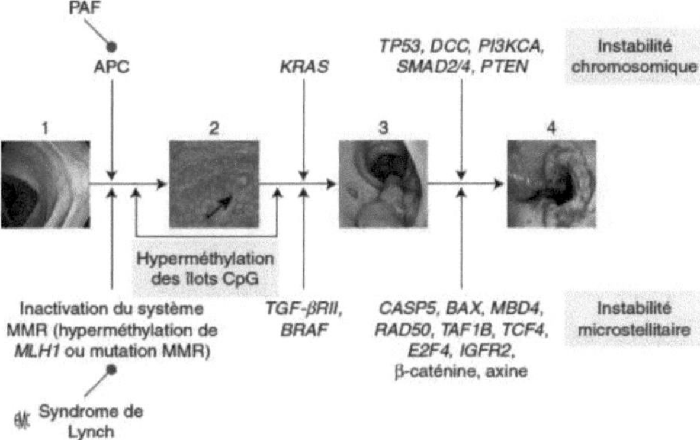


**Figure 14** Main molecular abnormalities according to carcinogenesis pathway : 1. Normal mucosa; 2. Aberrant crypts; 3. Adenomas; 4. Invasive cancer (42).

Adenomas are benign epithelial tumors whose growth is defined by loss of control over cell proliferation and varying degrees of dysplasia. There are four main histological types of adenoma. Tubular adenoma (around 75% of adenomas), villous adenoma and tubulovillous adenoma (46). They are associated with the CIN phenotype. A small adenoma may take six years to develop into an adenoma larger than 1 cm, and this adenoma may take around 17 years to develop into an adenocarcinoma, and then around two years to acquire the properties leading to metastatic dissemination (Fig.15) (47). The fourth type is the scalloped adenoma, featuring a scalloped (sawtooth) appearance with cellular atypia often corresponding to dysplastic lesions. Scalloped adenomas tend to be located in the right colon, occur preferentially in women, and are often multiple. They are associated with microsatellite instability and/or hypermethylation of CpG islets.
Colorectal carcinogenesis thus shows certain differences between the classical pathway of tubular adenoma transformation (CIN) and other pathways (48) (scalloped adenomas and MSI-H CRCs; flat dysplasia and IBD-associated CRCs).

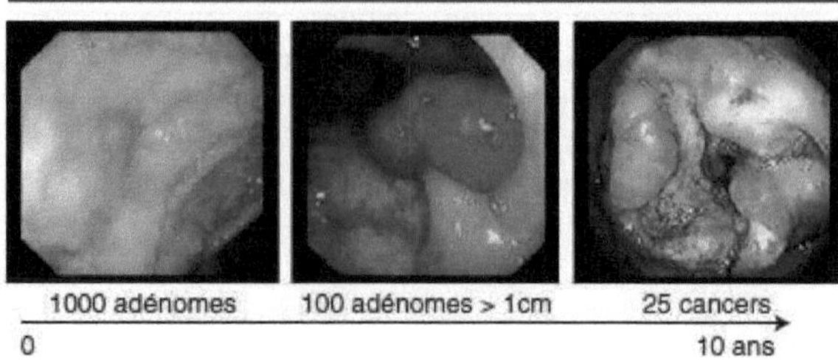


**Figure 15** Adenoma - colorectal cancer sequence (49).

## 3. Molecular basis of colorectal carcinogenesis :

The genetic instability of cancer cells explains why the tumor genome accumulates numerous alterations.

Among the genes involved in colorectal carcinogenesis, some are proto-oncogenes (*KRAS, β-catenin, BRAF*), others are tumor suppressor genes (*APC, TP53, DCC [deleted in colorectal carcinoma], SMAD4, SMAD2, TGF-βRII [TGF-β receptor type II], IGF2R [insulin-like growth factor 2 receptor], BAX [BCL2-associated X protein], MLH1, MSH2, PMS1, PMS2, MSH6, PTEN [phosphatase and tensin homolog]*). Proto-oncogenes code for proteins involved in signal transduction, acting directly or indirectly on the cell cycle. Their activation following gene alterations leads to continuous cell proliferation in the absence of growth signals, and modification of just one of the two alleles is sufficient to lead to a gain of function (50). Tumor suppressor genes, on the other hand, maintain genome integrity, including DNA repair, and inactivation of both alleles leads to the genetic instability necessary for tumor progression.

### *a) Chromosomal instability :*

Chromosomal instability (CIN) is found in approximately 75% of sporadic CRCs, but also in all patients with PAF. These tumors are preferentially located in the left colon and rectum. The CIN phenotype is characterized by abnormalities in chromosome number or structure, with gain or loss of whole chromosomes or chromosome segments leading to aneuploidy (loss of heterozygosity). The regions most frequently deleted in CRCs are chromosomes 5q, 8p, 17p, 18q and 22q.

Through the loss or gain of genetic material, chromosomal instability contributes to the inactivation of tumor suppressor genes and the activation of proto-oncogenes.

A number of tumor suppressor genes have been identified in these deleted regions, including *APC, TP53, DCC, Cables, SMAD2* and *SMAD4*.

Chromosomal instability can be observed in the early stages of carcinogenesis, as evidenced by the chromosomal loss observed in the majority of adenomas. In CIN tumours, the tumour process most often begins with an inactivating mutation of one of the genes in the Wnt/APC/β-catenin pathway (most often *APC*), followed by an activating mutation in the KRAS/BRAF pathway, promoting the growth of aberrant crypts and adenomatous lesions. Subsequently, inactivation of tumor suppressor genes such as *TP53* and alteration of other signaling pathways, such as *TGF-β* (*SMAD2* and *SMAD4*), *DCC, PI3KCA, PTEN* participate in the transformation of an adenoma into an adenocarcinoma (Fig.13, Fig.14).

### *b) Microsatellite instability :*

Microsatellite instability (MSI-H) is present in around 15% of sporadic CRCs, and in 95% of cases of Lynch syndrome or HNPCC (hereditary Non Polyposis Colon Cancer).

This is a particular form of genetic instability affecting the repeated sequences of the genome, the microsatellites, which are naturally more difficult to replicate. Microsatellite mismatches occur physiologically during replication, and are normally repaired by the MMR (Mis Match Repaire) system, consisting mainly of the MLH1, MSH2, MSH6 and PMS2 proteins.

MSI-H tumours are more often located in the right colon (less than 5% of left colon tumours are MSI-H, and over 90% of right colon tumours are MSI-H). They occur either at an early age (Lynch syndrome) or at a late age (sporadic cases). They are often poorly differentiated, with a significant mucosal colloid component. Unlike CIN tumors, these tumors rarely have mutations in *APC, KRAS* and *TP53*, and are diploid (Fig.13, Fig.14).

In contrast, *BRAF* mutation is frequently present in over 80% of MSI-H CRCs with *MLH1* hypermethylation. *TGF-βRII* (TGF-β type II receptor) and *BRAF* mutations are early events in these tumors. It is now accepted that sporadic MSI-H tumors derive from scalloped adenomas. This MSI-H phenotype is associated with a significant tumor lymphocyte infiltrate, as well as better survival after curative surgery. On the other hand, these tumors appear to be less sensitive to 5-fluorouracil (5-FU) (51).

### *c) Hypermethylation of CpG islets:*

Epigenetic modifications are a set of phenomena that influence the expression of a gene without modifying its DNA sequence. They can be transmitted during mitosis.

Hypermethylation of CpG islands is the most frequent epigenetic modification in cancer. CpG islands are regions rich in cytosine-guanine dinucleotides located at the promoters and first exons of genes. It is well established that methylation of a CpG island at the promoter is associated with transcriptional silencing of the gene concerned.

There is currently no consensus as to which markers should be used to determine the methylator phenotype or CIMP (*CpG island methylator phenotype*).

As with MSI-H CRCs, CIMP tumors develop predominantly from scalloped adenomas. The CIMP phenotype is found in around 20% to 30% of CRCs, and is associated with the MSI-H phenotype in around 50% to 60% of cases.

The CIMP phenotype is more frequent in tumors of the right colon, in poorly differentiated tumors and in women. The CIMP phenotype has been associated with a poor prognosis after curative surgery, but these tumors are thought to be sensitive to 5-FU.

In colorectal carcinogenesis, this phenomenon occurs early in precancerous cells of aberrant crypt foci, scalloped adenomas and large hyperplastic polyps.

### *d) CMS (Consensus Molecular System) molecular classification :*

Colorectal cancer is a highly heterogeneous group of diseases. Based on 6 molecular classifications and over 4000 patients, an international consortium of experts has recently identified 4 subtypes of colorectal cancer (52).
This is the CMS classification into 4 groups characterized by molecular, biological and clinical factors (53). It should be noted that 21% of CRCs do not belong to any of these 4 groups (Table 1).

**CMS-1 Group (MSI, Immune) :**
Represents 13% of CRCs and characterized by tumors with microsatellite instability (MSI high), marked immune infiltration, often CIMP high (CIMP high = methylator phenotype) and BRAF-mutated tumors. Preferentially located on the right. Their prognosis is good in the absence of metastasis, and poor in the event of metastatic progression (poor survival after relapse).
**CMS-2 Group (Canonical) :**
Represents 35% of left-sided CRCs without microsatellite instability (MSS), marked by frequent somatic mutations (SCNA high) with frequent EGFR overexpression and activation of the WNT/MYC pathway.
Their prognosis is intermediate.
**Group CMS-3 (Metabolic)** :
Represents 11% of CRCs, of epithelial type, MSS in 90% of cases, and characterized by frequent RAS mutations and few somatic mutations. They are distributed fairly evenly between the left and right colon. Their prognosis is intermediate.
**Group CMS-4 (Mesenchymal) :**
Represents 20% of CRCs. They are characterized by numerous somatic alterations (SCNA high), frequent activation of TGFß and angiogenesis, tumors more often MSI, and are located preferentially in the left colon. Their prognosis is poor in metastatic situations.

**Table 1** Molecular classification of CRCs (Consensus Molecular System) (53).

| CMS1 MSI immune | CMS2 Canonical | CMS3 Metabolic | CMS4 Mesenchymal |
|---|---|---|---|
| 14% | 37% | 13% | 23% |
| MSI, CIMP high, hypermutation | SCNA high | Mixed MSI status, SCNA low, CIMP low | SCNA high |
| *BRAF* mutations | | *KRAS* mutations | |
| Immune infiltration and activation | WNT and MYC activation | Metabolic deregulation | Stromal infiltration, TGF-β activation, angiogenesis |
| Worse survival after relapse | | | Worse relapse-free and overall survival |

# III. Anatomical reminder :

## A. Anatomy of the colon:

The colon, or large intestine, lies between the small intestine and the rectum. For the surgeon, it comprises two main sections: the right colon, vascularized by branches of the superior mesenteric artery, and the left colon, vascularized by the inferior mesenteric artery. It forms a frame (Fig.16) in the abdominal cavity, and in its various segments, enters into successive relationships with almost all intra-abdominal viscera.

A distinction must be made between contiguous colonic segments (ascending and descending) and mobile segments (transverse and sigmoid) linked by a long free meso (Fig.17).

The transverse mesocolon divides the abdominal cavity into two distinct levels, supra- and sub-mesocolic. The mesosigmoid isolates the lesser pelvis (54).

### Vascularization :

Colonic arteries are derived from the superior and inferior mesenteric arteries. Up to and including the middle third of the transverse colon, the colon is vascularized by the ileocolic artery and the right colic artery, collateral branches of the right edge of the superior mesenteric artery.

The cecum is vascularized by the anterior and posterior cecal arteries, terminal branches of the ileocolic artery. The appendix is vascularized by the appendicular artery, which arises from the posterior caecal artery. The appendicular lymph nodes drain into the ileocolic lymph nodes.

The rest of the colon is vascularized by the left colic artery and the trunk of the sigmoid arteries, collateral branches of the inferior mesenteric artery.

Each colonic artery gives rise to an upper and lower branch which, when anastomosed, form a vascular arcade bordering the colon, from the ileocolic artery to the inferior sigmoid artery. Two inconstant branches of the superior mesenteric artery sometimes complete the vascularization of the colon: the middle colic artery between the ileocolic artery and the right colic artery for the ascending colon, and the colica media artery between the right and left colic arteries for the transverse colon (Fig.18).

The veins, satellites of the arteries, drain into the inferior and superior mesenteric veins, then the portal vein.

Lymphatic drainage takes place via lymph nodes along the arteries to their origin. They are divided into five groups: epicolic (in contact with the intestinal wall), paracolic (in contact with the bordering arch), intermediate (along the pedicles), main (at the origin of the colonic branches on the mesenteric artery) and central (periaorto-caval, at the posterior surface of the head of the pancreas).

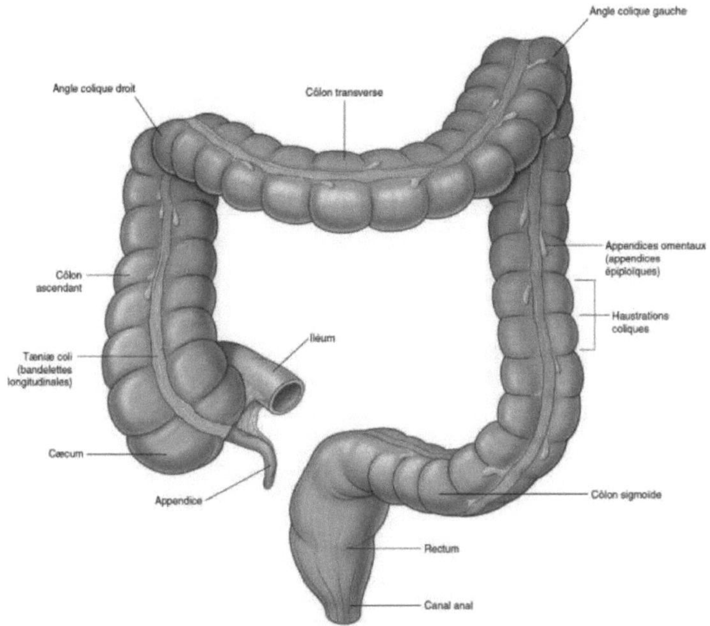


**Figure 16** External morphology of the colon (55).

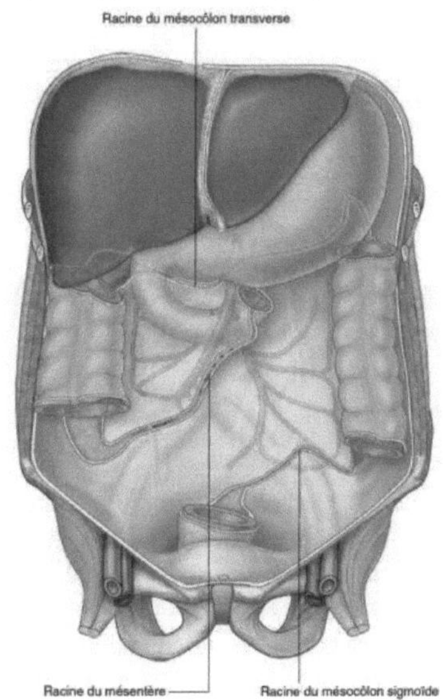


**Figure 17** Peritoneal reflections on the posterior abdominal wall (55).

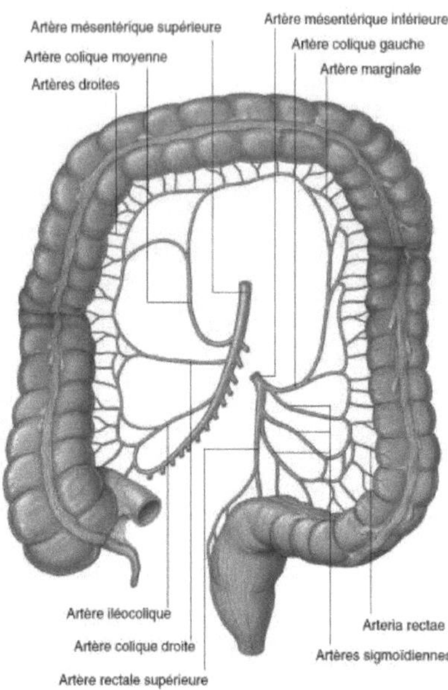


**Figure 18** Arterial vascularization of the colon (55).

## Surgical interest :

In open surgery, exploration of the entire colonic framework requires a wide approach: long median or transverse. A laparoscopic approach can also be used, enabling the external morphology of mobile colonic segments to be followed. Fixed segments, as in open surgery, can only be explored after coloparietal detachment. The laparoscopic approach does not allow any lesions to be palpated. Whatever the approach, the most difficult region to explore reliably is the left angular region.

Operative exposure of the colon is more or less easy depending on the morphology of the subject: it can be laborious in the obese, with short, thick and fragile mesos and a "lipomatous" omentum.

## B. Anatomy of the rectum :

### 1. External morphology :

The rectum follows the sigmoid colon. It is molded onto the sacral concavity, median and globally vertical in a frontal plane, hence its name (*rectum* in Latin means straight). It begins opposite S3, and lacks a band, haustration and omental appendage, which differentiates it from the colon. 15 cm long, the rectum has an upper part covered with visceral peritoneum (peritoneal part) and a non-peritoneal part (sub-peritoneal part).

The rectum can be divided into three parts according to the distance from the pectineal line (or upper edge of the sphincter):

-The lower rectum, less than 2 cm from the upper edge of the sphincter, i.e. less than 5 cm from the anal margin;
-The middle rectum, extending from 2 to 7 cm from the upper edge of the sphincter, i.e. from 5 to 10 cm from the anal margin;
-The upper rectum, extended more than 7 cm from the upper edge of the sphincter, i.e. 10 to 15 cm from the anal margin (Fig.19).

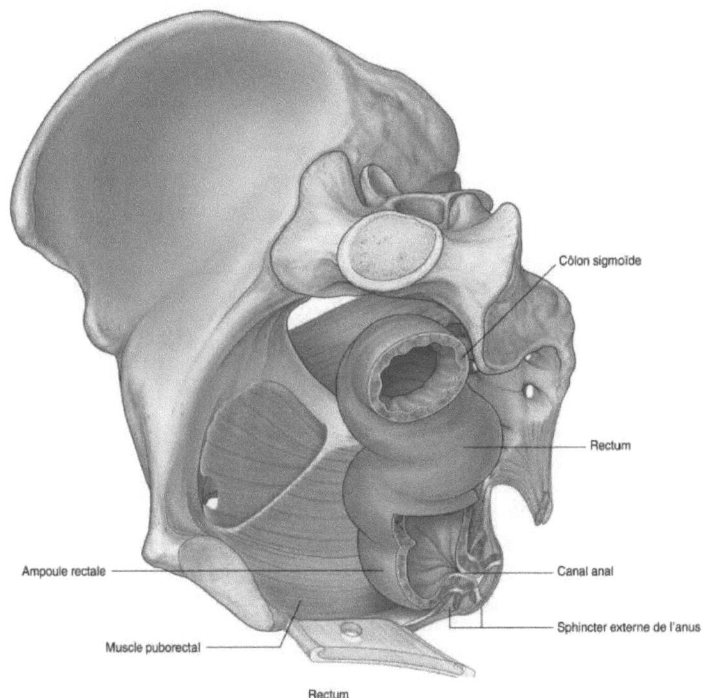


**Figure 19** Rectum and anal canal (55).

## 2. **Reports :**

The subperitoneal rectum is located within a fibrous lodge formed by four walls. The cellulo-lymphatic tissue surrounding the rectum within the loge is called the mesorectum. The word "mesorectum" does not exist in the "Gray's Anatomy" index or the "Terminologia Anatomica" of anatomists, it was described by a surgeon R.J Heald (56).

The mesorectum is developed over three quarters of the circumference of the subperitoneal rectum, posteriorly and laterally up to 2-3 cm from the anorectal junction (Fig.20). The anterior surface of the subperitoneal rectum and the last 2-3 cm of the pelvic rectum are usually devoid of fatty tissue. The mesorectum is surrounded by a thin but still individualizable envelope known as the visceral sheet of pelvic fascia or fascia recti.

The pelvic walls are covered by the parietal layer of this pelvic fascia, which corresponds posteriorly to the presacral fascia (Waldeyer's fascia). This parietal fascia covers the pelvic vessels and nerve branches of the superior (sympathetic) and inferior (parasympathetic) hypogastric plexuses, and the ureters. Between these two layers, visceral and parietal, there is an avascular sliding space, mainly present posteriorly.

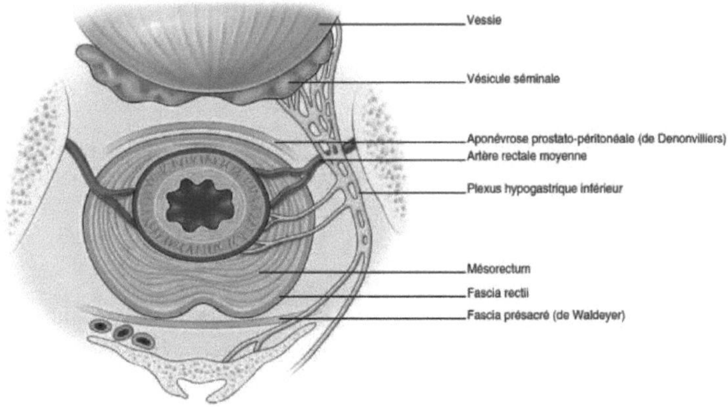


**Figure 20** Male mesorectum (55).

The two leaflets symphysis posteriorly and anteriorly below the cul-de-sac of Douglas. In front, they form the prostatoperitoneal aponeurosis of Denonvilliers in men, and the rectovaginal septum in women. In front of the Denonvilliers aponeurosis runs the cavernous nerve, which arises from the lateral pelvic plexus and runs to the posterolateral surface of the prostate, accompanied by the capsular artery, forming Walsh's neurovascular bands. At this level, the cavernous nerve is very close to the anterolateral aspect of the lower rectum. Posteriorly, opposite the fourth sacral piece, 3 or 4 cm from the anorectal junction, the two sheets fuse to form the rectosacral ligament. Veins emerge from the presacral holes (presacral veins), exactly where the rectosacral ligament attaches. Laterally, beneath the peritoneum, there are fibrous adhesions between the visceral and parietal sheets, called the lateral ligaments (formerly known as the rectal fins), which represent a point of lateral attachment of the mesorectum to the lateral pelvic wall. These lateral ligaments accompany the anorectal nerves of the inferior hypogastric plexus. Apart from these few branches, the lateral pelvic nerves and plexuses do not penetrate the mesorectum. Branches of the parasympathetic system originating from the S2, S3 and S4 roots (erector nerves), which join the lateral pelvic plexus, run beneath the parietal sheet represented by the pyramidal fascia. At the level of the lateral ligaments, the middle rectal artery is very inconstant.

## 3. Vascularization :

### *a) Arteries :*

Arterial vascularization is ensured mainly by the superior rectal artery, and more secondarily by the middle and inferior rectal arteries and the median sacral artery.

### *b) Veins :*

Venous vascularization of the rectum is quite similar to arterial vascularization. It is ensured essentially by the superior rectal vein, and secondarily by the inferior and middle rectal veins and the median sacral vein.

### *c) Lymph nodes :*

Lymphatic vessels form from lymphatic plexuses in the rectal wall beneath the rectal and anal mucosa. They then reach the perirectal lymph nodes located in the mesorectum. Lymphatic drainage of the rectum is satellite to the arteries, and for most of the rectum takes place in the mesorectum, ascending to the inferior mesenteric artery via the superior rectal artery. Lymphatics draining the perineal rectum and anorectal junction can go laterally to perineal structures via the sphincters and levator muscles, but also upwards outside the fascia recti, and much more rarely to the internal iliac vessels. Thus, lymphatic drainage is mainly towards the superior rectal pedicle through the mesorectum, and secondarily towards the internal or external iliac lymph nodes and the inguinal lymph nodes by following the pudendal and subcutaneous lymphatic networks.

## 4. Innervation :

The pelvic parts of the prevertebral plexuses carry sympathetic, parasympathetic and visceral afferent fibers (Fig.21). The pelvic parts of the plexuses are responsible for innervation of the pelvic viscera and erectile tissues of the perineum. The prevertebral plexuses enter the pelvis in the form of two hypogastric nerves, one on each side, which cross the upper pelvic opening medial to the internal iliac vessels. The hypogastric nerves arise from the superior hypogastric plexus, which lies anterior to the L5 vertebra between the promontory of the sacrum and the bifurcation of the aorta. In men, the superior hypogastric plexus is responsible for ejaculation.

When the hypogastric nerves are joined by the pelvic splanchnic nerves carrying preganglionic parasympathetic fibers from S2 to S4, the lateral pelvic plexuses (inferior hypogastric plexuses) are formed. The lower hypogastric plexuses, one on each side, run down the pelvic walls, medial to the large vessels and somatic nerves. They give rise to the following subsidiary plexuses innervating the pelvic viscera: rectal plexus, uterovaginal plexus, prostatic plexus and bladder plexus. The terminal branches of the lower hypogastric plexuses penetrate and cross the deep space of the perineum, and innervate the erectile tissues of the penis and clitoris in the perineum. In men, these nerves are called the cavernous nerves.

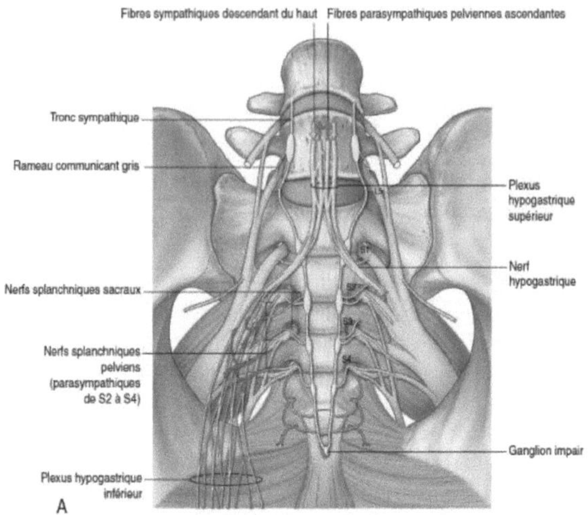


**Figure 21** Pelvic extensions of the prevertebral plexuses (55).

## C. Liver anatomy :

### 1. External morphology

The liver weighs around 2% of body weight (on average 1.5 kg). Its density is estimated at 1, which makes it possible to evaluate its volume.

It is located in the supra-mesocolic region, in the right hypochondrium and part of the epigastrium, under the right diaphragmatic dome and part of the left.

Asymmetrical ovoid, highly developed on the right, it has a large transverse axis, measuring around 28 cm wide, 8 cm high and 16 cm from front to back.

Three edges are described (including the ventral anterior edge, which is thin and sometimes palpable under the costal margin), and three faces (diaphragmatic, dorsal visceral, caudal visceral) (Fig.22) :

The diaphragmatic side is convex (the dome), smooth and follows the shape of the diaphragm, and is divided by the insertion of the falciform ligament;

The visceral side (Fig.23) (divided into a caudal anterior part and a dorsal posterior part):

The caudal visceral surface is irregular and marked by three grooves:

-The left sulcus, formed by the fissure of the round ligament in front of the hepatic hilum and by the venous ligament behind it,

-The right sulcus, formed by the vesicular bed that joins the anterior edge of the liver to the hepatic hilum,

-The transverse sulcus, formed by the hilum that joins the right and left sulci.

We thus define the left lobe medial to the left sulcus, the right lobe lateral to the right sulcus, and between these two sulci the square lobe anterior to the transverse sulcus and the caudate lobe posterior to it.

The dorsal visceral surface is vertical, marked laterally by a wide vertical sulcus sometimes completely surrounding the inferior vena cava, and medially by the sulcus of the venous ligament (Arantius sulcus). The two sulci delimit the caudate lobe (Spiegel's lobe). A large part of this face is devoid of peritoneum between the peritoneal reflection lines, forming the coronary ligament.

Two main lobes are described externally, bounded by the insertion of the round ligament and the falciform ligament, the left sulcus and the sulcus of the venous ligament: the right lobe (around 75% of volume) and the left lobe (around 25% of volume). On the caudal visceral side, we describe the square lobe between the hilum, umbilical fissure and vesicular fossa, and the caudate lobe between the hilum and sulcus of the venous ligament.

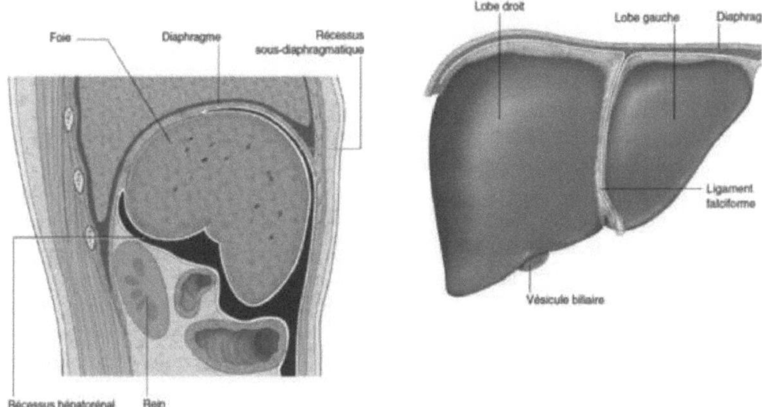


**Figure 22** Liver faces and associated liver recesses (55).

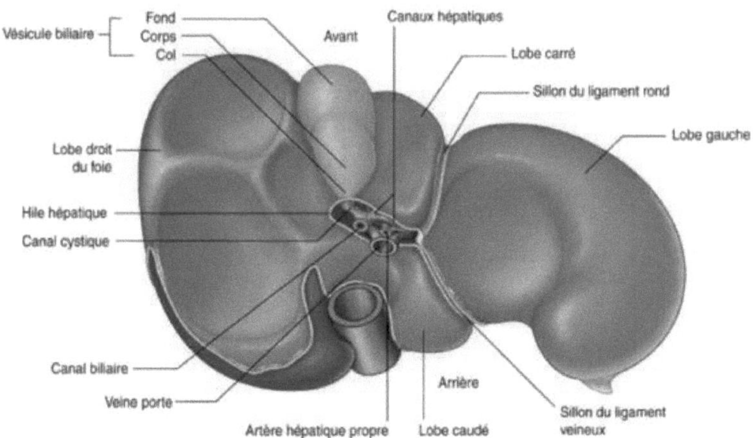


**Figure 23** Visceral surfaces of the liver (55).

## 2. **Fixity, ligaments :**

The liver is attached to the diaphragm and posterior wall by the broad coronary ligament, centered on the diaphragm's vena cava and extending laterally to the thinner right and left triangular ligaments. The liver is closely attached to the inferior vena cava by its adventitia and the hepatic veins. The small omentum inserts into the groove of the venous ligament.

## 3. **Reports :**

The caudal visceral surface of the liver responds: on the right, to the right kidney, the genu superiorus, and the right colonic angle; on the left, to the stomach, and sometimes to the upper pole of the spleen.

The posterior visceral side responds to the retrohepatic portion of the inferior vena cava, the posterior insertions and right pillar of the diaphragm, and the esophagus.

## 4. **Vascularization :**

The liver has two vascular pedicles: a lower afferent or hepatic pedicle and an upper efferent venous pedicle.

The inferior afferent pedicle, or hepatic pedicle, is distinctive for its double vascularization, arterial (proper hepatic artery (Fig.24), dividing into right and left hepatic arteries) and venous (portal vein). The hepatic arteries and portal vein enter the liver through the hilum, with the portal vein behind and the hepatic arteries in front and to the left.

The superior venous efferent pedicle consists of the three main hepatic veins: left, middle and right, which drain into the inferior vena cava at the posterosuperior edge of the liver. Part of the hepatic venous blood flows directly into the retrohepatic inferior vena cava via accessory hepatic veins arising from adjacent hepatic segments. Liver lymph nodes are located on both sides of the inferior afferent pedicle.

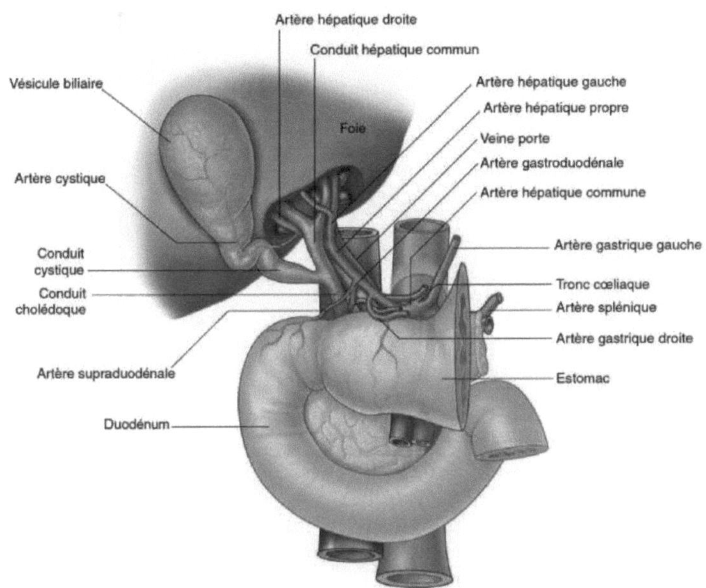


**Figure 24** Afferent vascularization of the liver (55).

## 5. **Internal morphology and segmentation :**

Claude Couinaud, a French surgeon and anatomist, described the segmentation of the liver, based on the intrahepatic distribution of the portal vein, on which the arterial and biliary distributions are modelled (Fig.25). This segmentation is determined by virtual planes. A right and a left liver are thus distinguished, separated by the main (virtual) scissural plane and corresponding to the two bifurcation branches of the portal vein. On the right, the short right branch divides into an anterior (or paramedian, anterior sector) and a posterior (or lateral, posterior sector) branch, each of which divides into an inferior and an upper branch, thus defining the four right segments: V, VIII, VI and VII. On the left, the long left portal branch divides into a lateral branch (segment II) and a paramedian branch (segments III and IV, separated by the umbilical scissure, with the underside of segment IV corresponding to the square lobe). The dorsal sector, corresponding to segment I or Spiegel's caudate lobe, depends on small portal branches coming from the dorsal face of the portal bifurcation.

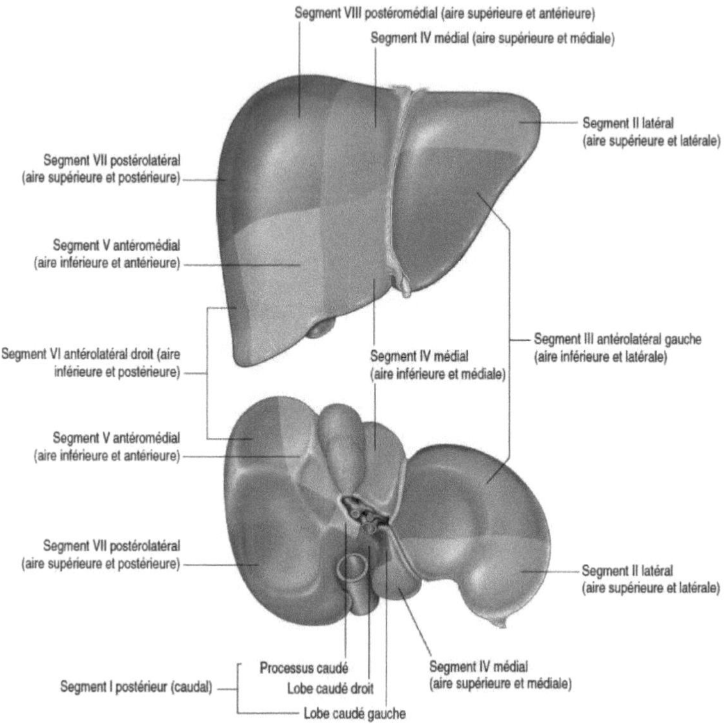


**Figure 25** Liver segmentation according to Couinaud (55).

The hepatic arteries, portal vein and bile ducts are surrounded in their intrahepatic course by a fibrous sheath corresponding to a thickening of the liver capsule that penetrates the parenchyma at the hilum, forming a sort of fibrous skeleton (hilar plate).

# IV. Pathological anatomy:

Pathological anatomy is a changing discipline in digestive pathology. Its traditional role, through morphological analysis of cells and tissues, is to diagnose or help diagnose disease. Similarly, prognostic assessment is still based, when a patient undergoes surgery, on an appreciation of the locoregional evolutionary stage of the disease. A major advance in this field has been the almost universal adoption of the pTNM system of cancer classification.
In addition to this "traditional" role, pathological anatomy is now involved at every stage in the management of patients with colorectal cancer:
-Prevention and screening, by studying lesions discovered during screening colonoscopies.
-Epidemiology through the production of data that can be transmitted to tumor registries and other public bodies.
Above all, therapeutic management: this involves the indication of adjuvant treatments, either chemotherapy, whose indication is often based on the pTNM stage, or, more recently, "targeted therapies" guided by the characteristics of the tumor, generally assessed by the in situ detection of genetic abnormalities or the expression of certain proteins. (57).

## 1. Main precancerous tissue lesion :

### *Adenoma:*

For both types of colorectal cancer (chromosomal instability / microsatellite instability), it is currently accepted that most cancers develop from a precancerous tumor lesion: the adenoma.
There is a sequence of normal mucosal transformation → adenoma → adenocarcinoma by accumulation of genetic alterations involving oncogenes and tumor suppressor genes (58). Macroscopically, the adenoma corresponds to a polyp (sessile or pedunculated), protruding into the colonic lumen. More rarely, it is a flat adenoma defined by an adenomatous lesion less than twice the height of the normal mucosa, corresponding macroscopically to a rough or erythematous area that is difficult to see endoscopically.
An adenoma is a benign glandular epithelial tumor. By definition, colonic adenomas are always dysplastic, corresponding to a circumscribed focus of dysplastic epithelium. Adenomas are classified according to their endoscopic appearance (sessile, pedicled, planar); microscopic architecture (tubular: more than 80% tubes; tubulo-cultivated, villous: more than 80% villi) and degree of dysplasia (low grade, high grade).
Not all adenomas inevitably lead to cancer. It is estimated that only 10% of adenomas reach 1 cm or more. Overall, only 1/4 of adenomas over 1 cm will become cancerous.
Transformation of an adenoma into an adenocarcinoma takes an estimated 10 to 20 years, which may be shorter in the case of MSI+ adenomas.

## 2. Topography of the ACC :

The majority of CRCs occur in the sigmoid and rectum, although a different trend, with a greater proportion in the proximal colon, has been observed in recent years. Molecular studies have shown topographical differences according to the molecular profile of CRCs. MSI-H CRCs and those with RAS mutations are more often located in the cecum, ascending colon and transverse colon.

## 3. Macroscopy :

Macroscopic aspects are influenced by the natural history of these tumours, colonic diameter and stool consistency (faecal dehydration favours ulceration). On the right, cancers are vegetative and exophytic, not very ulcerated, often very large. In the transverse and descending colons, which are narrow in diameter, a ferrule is rapidly formed. In the rectum, they most frequently form a ring around a central ulceration. A distinction is thus made between :

### (1) Vegetable shapes :

These are sessile exophytic masses, protruding into the colonic lumen, often villeous in appearance, often eroded on the surface.

### (2) Ulcero-infiltrating forms:

They are made up of an ulceration surrounded by a roughly circular extension, and thus constitute the ferrule which can reach the entire circumference, leading to stenosis of the lumen.

### (3) Mixed forms :

They are common.

### (4) Plastic linoleum :

They form a thickened, rigid segment several centimetres long.

## 4. Histopathology:

The WHO classification identifies several histological types (59).

***a) Adenocarcinomas:*** Adenocarcinomas account for almost 95% of CRCs.

### *b) Particular histological forms :*

- Mucinous adenocarcinoma (mucinous colloid): Represents 10-15% of colorectal adenocarcinomas, defined by the presence of more than 50% of the mucinous component, the macroscopic appearance is gelatinous colloid, histologically they are made up of broad patches of pale mucinous substance containing distended and sometimes ruptured glandular tubes, cell trabeculae and isolated "kitten-ring" cells.

Kitten-ring cell carcinoma: also known as single-cell carcinoma or independent-cell carcinoma, it is rare, accounting for around 1% of CRCs, and should be investigated for possible gastric kitten-ring cell carcinoma. The tumor infiltrates the wall, relatively sparing the mucosa, which accounts for the frequent negativity of biopsies; these carcinomas more often infiltrate the peritoneum and ovaries.

-Undifferentiated carcinoma: Rare tumor showing no particular differentiation and presenting a variety of histological aspects. This category includes medullary carcinoma.
-Squamous cell carcinoma: Consisting solely of squamous cells, it is rare and has a poor prognosis.
-Adeno-squamous carcinoma: Defined by the presence of numerous squamous foci, either interspersed with or separate from the adenocarcinomatous component, the prognosis is also poorer than that of adenocarcinoma.
Small-cell carcinoma: morphologically, immunohistochemically and evolutionarily similar to small-cell carcinoma of the lung, it is often diagnosed at the stage of dissemination, in which case surgery is contraindicated.
-Other rare forms of CRC :
Spindle cell carcinoma,
Giant cell carcinoma,
Choriocarcinoma,
Pigmented carcinoma,
Clear cell carcinoma,
Stem cell carcinoma,
Carcinoma rich in Paneth cells (cryptic cell carcinoma),
Mixed carcinomas,
Scalloped adenocarcinoma: This is a variety of adenocarcinoma characterized by a scalloped architecture, accounting for 5.5% of CRCs and 17.5% of proximal CRCs; it develops on scalloped polyps. Its prognosis is poorer when it is of MSI phenotype (-) and distal location (60),
Micropapillary adenocarcinoma: poor prognosis.

### *c) Grading :*

It is based on the percentage of glands according to the WHO 2010 grading criteria, and distinguishes: (table 2)

**Table 2** WHO 2010 histological classification (grading) (61).

| Critère | Catégorie de différenciation | N° du Grade [a] | Description du Grade |
|---|---|---|---|
| >95% avec formation de glande | Bien différencié | 1 | Faible |
| 50-95% avec formation de glande | Moyennement différencié | 2 | Faible |
| >0-49% avec formation de glande | peu différencié | 3 | Elevée |
| Haut degré d'instabilité microsatellite [b] | Variable | Variable | Faible |

[a] La catégorie « carcinome indifférencié » (Grade 4) est réservée aux carcinomes Sans structure glandulaire, sans production de mucine ou aux carcinomes présentant une différenciation neuroendocrine squameuses ou sarcomatoïde.
[b] MSI-H.

Traditional WHO grading was based on four grades (good, moderate, poorly differentiated, undifferentiated) and a semi-quantitative assessment of the percentage of glands present. The 2010 WHO version (59) is based on two grades, with well and moderately differentiated grades grouped as low grade, and poorly differentiated and undifferentiated grades grouped as high grade. This assessment must also take into account two other parameters: histological type and MSI molecular status.

### d) *Tumor stroma :*

It may be inflammatory, consisting of a more or less marked lymphocytic infiltrate, or even of lymphoid follicles (Crohn-like), and may be observed within and/or around the tumor. These aspects are particularly noticeable in MSI+ tumors.

### e) *Immunophenotype :*

Primary and/or metastatic CRCs can be differentiated from other carcinomas by expression: ACE (+), β-catenin (nuclear labeling +), cytokeratin 20 (+), and negativity for cytokeratin7, CDX2 is useful to distinguish them from non-intestinal carcinomas, note that sporadic MSI (+) CRCs may not express CK20 or β-catenin.

## 5. Extension and evolution :

### a) *Locoregional extension :*

The cancer progresses locally, invading the various layers of the colorectal wall, the peritoneum and neighbouring organs. It reaches the entire circumference of the intestine in about two years (1/4 circumference every 6 months).
- Extension through the different layers of the wall :
Intraepithelial carcinoma: Difficult to distinguish from severe dysplasia, there is no rupture of the basement membrane.
Intramucosal cancer: the basement membrane is ruptured and the chorion invaded. There is a risk of venous invasion, given the presence of vessels in the chorion, but the probability of lymph node metastasis is nil at this stage.
Extension to the sub-mucosa: at this stage, there is a risk of lymphatic invasion: this is minimal in the case of superficial extension of the polyp axis, and reaches 27% in the case of extension to the colonic sub-mucosa.
The various layers of the wall are then reached.
-Transverse extension leads to a circular tumor responsible for obstructive stenosis
-Microscopic longitudinal extension above and below the tumour occurs mainly in the submucosa, rarely exceeding 2cm in rectal resections. A distal safety margin of 2cm is required.
-Regional extension is to the peritoneum and to neighbouring organs through contiguity from near to near, but also through distant grafts. In 50% to 75% of cases, macroscopic invasion or adhesion to a neighbouring organ corresponds to histological tumour invasion.
Depending on its location, CRC can invade various neighboring organs.
In rectal cancer, distal microscopic progression may be observed in the mesorectum up to 3-4cm beyond the lower pole of the tumour, without intra-parietal tumour extension. It occurs in 10-20% of cases, and justifies excision of the entire mesorectum.
Lateral spread towards the pelvic wall is most common in tumours of the lower rectum. Measurement of this lateral tumour extension is defined by lateral

clearance: this is the distance in millimetres between the zone of maximum tumour extension and the surgical section. If this distance is less than 1mm, tumour invasion of the radial margin is considered to have occurred, and the resection is considered to be of type R1.
The presence of emboli in peritumoral veins or lymphatics is found in 50% of cases. Venous invasion is predictive of the development of liver metastases.
Local extension may also occur along the nerves, and is found in 30% to 60% of excised specimens, and is a poor prognostic factor.

### b) *Invasion of lymph nodes :*

Invasion of lymph nodes from the tumor onwards occurs from proximal to proximal. Lymphatic vessels are satellites of arterial pedicles.
In principle, lymph node invasion is continuous, progressive and anatomical, and does not skip relays. It is related to the degree of parietal infiltration of the tumor, but also to its degree of differentiation; poorly differentiated forms metastasize early.
However, in less than 5% of cases, skip-metastases can be observed. These are metastases that bypass one or more lymph node relays to reach the pedicle nodes directly.
In colorectal cancers, it occurs first in the peri-tumoral lymph nodes, then in the intermediate lymph nodes and those at the origin of the vascular pedicles.
In the case of rectal tumors, lymphatic extension occurs in the mesorectum and then along the satellite lymph nodes of the branches of the inferior mesenteric artery. Excision of the mesorectum and curage of the inferior mesenteric lymph nodes are therefore necessary.
Assessment of lymph node status in CRC requires examination of at least 12 nodes according to (UICC) (62).

### c) *Hematogenous metastases :*

In ¾ of cases, metastases occur first in the liver, then in the lung and then in other organs. Venous invasion is observed in half of all cases. The right liver is more often invaded than the left.

## 6. Anatomopathological report :

All the criteria on a typical pathology report are macroscopic, histological, immunohistochemical and molecular. (63).

### a) *Macroscopic examination :*

It is carried out in the pathology department, in conjunction with the surgeon if necessary. It covers the conditioning of the surgical specimen (in particular the type of fixator used) and its precise description. This includes the length of the specimen, its size, the distance between the tumour and the nearest resection limit, the appearance of the tumour, the percentage of circumferential invasion, whether or not a perforation has been confirmed in the tumour zone, the presence of nodules of carcinosis and other possible lesions, and the appearance of the mesorectum. The latter is essential for assessing the quality of surgical excision of this anatomical structure. In practice, it is based on the determination of three grades according to Quirke et al (64) (table 3 ). This classification reflects the quality of the surgery performed, which is closely linked to the risk of recurrence. Incomplete exeresis is in fact a source of local relapse, explained by microscopic tumour deposits left in place in the incompletely resected mesorectum.

It is recommended that photos be taken and included in the final report, to objectively document this macroscopic assessment.

**Table 3** Quirke classification.

| | Full (grade 3) | Almost complete (grade 2) | Incomplete (grade 1) |
|---|---|---|---|
| Appearance of the mesorectum | Intact, smooth | Moderately thick, irregular | Thin |
| Mesorectal wound | <5 mm | >5 mm and muscularis not visible | Visible muscles |
| Cone effect | Absent | Moderate | Present |
| Circumferential resection margin | Smooth, even | Irregular | Irregular |

**Macroscopic examination of liver metastasis :**

Macroscopic management must be rigorous and based on procedures that everyone can use. The aim is to identify the metastasis(es) present, and to match them with imaging data. This macroscopic stage must be based on accurate sampling of the lesions detected. Insufficient sampling can lead to over- or under-estimation of the response. In this context, it may be advisable to include all metastatic nodules smaller than 1 cm, and to take one sample per cm from lesions larger than 1 cm. A description of the number and size of lesions present should be included in the macroscopic report. It is also necessary to evaluate the surgical margin, after prior inking, from the nearest metastasis. This macroscopically assessed margin will be confirmed histologically on the samples taken opposite. This is an important parameter, as it influences the occurrence of recurrence. In addition to sampling the tumour lesions, it is useful to take a sample from the non-tumourous liver at a distance, to allow analysis of any liver toxicity associated with the chemotherapies used.

### *b) Microscopic examination :*

The microscopic elements that make up a report are varied. Some are unanimously recognized as prognostic, while others are promising but not yet validated for use in clinical practice. Microscopic examination must follow a precise procedure to ensure that no important parameter is omitted.

This is where the notion of a checklist comes into its own, as it must specify the histological type and grade of differentiation. The depth of extension (or level of infiltration) is determined from histological examination of a rigorously sampled CRC surgical specimen, and is classified according to the latest version of the pTNM classification. In this context, the prefix "p" stands for pathology, indicating that the TNM classification is based on pathological rather than clinical criteria.

In the case of neoadjuvant treatment, whether radiotherapy, chemotherapy, targeted therapy or their combination, the prefix "y" is added. Preoperative treatment of locally advanced or metastatic cancer may be accompanied by a cellular response in the primary tumor or metastatic site, in line with the efficacy of the treatment. This histological response can be assessed semi-quantitatively using different classifications, by evaluating the percentage of residual cells and regression, in the form of fibrosis or acellular colloid patches. Dworak's classification is one of the oldest (65).

Rectal cancer regression grade RCRG and mRCRG (modified RCRG) classifications are often used to assess therapeutic response at rectal level. Rubbia Brandt's TRG tumor regression grade classification is used to assess response in liver metastases (66) .

Morphological aspect of the infiltrative front: Colorectal cancers, mostly adenocarcinomas, can be characterized by either an "expansile" or "infiltrative" type of invasion. The infiltrative type has a poorer prognosis than the expansive type. It should be emphasized that the "expansive" type is more frequently found in cancers with MSI. Criteria have been proposed to distinguish between these two types of infiltration. In favor of the infiltrative type are the following: inability to distinguish the invasive front with the naked eye; inability to distinguish tumor tissue from stroma reaction with the naked eye; dissection of the muscularis without associated stroma reaction; and infiltration of pericolic adipose tissue by small glands, clusters or irregular trabeculae of tumor cells.

The morphological aspect of the invasion front has not been formally validated for prognostic use in clinical practice. This item is therefore optional in the pathology report.

Tumor budding: in the literal sense of the term, corresponds to the presence of isolated tumor cells or tumor clusters not exceeding five cells, at the tumor invasion front (67). This morphological aspect is more often associated with an "infiltrative" than an "expansive" invasion front. The spindle-shaped appearance of the tumor cells observed suggests that these lesions may be part of the epithelial-mesenchymal transition phenomenon, during which epithelial cells lose their morphological and phenotypic attributes and become candidates for local or distant dissemination. This item is optional in the pathology report.

Stroma lymphocyte response: Incrementing the intratumoral and peritumoral lymphocyte response (or Crohn-like response) on the pathological report of CRC may be useful for several reasons. On the one hand, it could allow morphological screening of strong host-related immune responses, whose favorable prognostic impact has been emphasized. On the other hand, an intratumoral lymphocytic infiltrate and a Crohn's-like reaction represent morphological criteria suggestive of MSI. This evaluation remains optional.

Surgical resection limits: The integrity or invasiveness of the proximal and distal surgical resection limits must be mentioned. For rectal tumors in non-peritoneal areas, the circumferential margin or clearance must be specified. This can be measured from the tumor or the nearest tumor structure, such as a metastatic lymph node or tumor deposit. The measurement of the circumferential resection margin corresponds to the distance between the area of deepest tumour infiltration and the resection limit of the previously inked mesorectum. Circumferential margin involvement is considered negative if the tumor is located more than 1 mm from the inked surface, and positive if the tumor is located less than 1 mm (63).

**Microscopy of liver metastasis:**

Conventional data :

Naturally, this assessment is intended to confirm the diagnosis of metastatic disease associated with colorectal adenocarcinoma. But it also corresponds to the estimation of histological response, reflecting the impact of induction treatment, whose prognostic role has been evoked. Analysis of this response or tumour "regression" is usually semi-quantitative (68). In practice, this analysis integrates the proportion of residual tumour cells and the proportion of regression in the form of fibrosis, necrosis or, much more rarely, colloid response. Several evaluation systems exist, based on publications that have demonstrated their prognostic impact. The most widely used classification is that of Rubbia-Brandt et al. (66) which was inspired by a five-grade classification proposed by Mandard et al. (69) in esophageal cancers initially treated with radio-chemotherapy. This histological classification, termed *Tumor Regression Grade* (TRG), ranges from metastases without any regression (TRG5) to sterilized metastases (TRG1), with intermediates including a variable proportion of residual tumor cells (TRG2: almost complete response with rare tumor cells associated with fibrosis, TRG3: partial response with more tumor cells, but predominantly fibrosis and TRG4: minimal response with tumor cells predominating over fibrosis). Based on these five grades, Rubbia-Brandt et al. defined three categories: major response (TRG1 and 2), partial response (TRG3) and minimal or absent response (TRG4 and 5), the first category having the best survival, the second an intermediate survival and the third the worst.

Emerging data :

In quantitative terms, measurement of the thickness of the peripheral residual tumor crown, located at the interface with the normal liver, could correlate with radiological and histological responses and have a prognostic impact (70). According to the authors, this measurement should be taken from the densest tumor territory at cellular level. These data were obtained from patients treated mainly with chemotherapy and Bevacizumab. They may reflect a better translation of the responses observed with biotherapies. However, the prognostic significance and reproducibility of this new quantitative criterion remain to be confirmed in complementary series.

With regard to qualitative aspects, a work by Mentha (71) has shown that the morphological presentation of residual tumor remnants can also have a clinical impact. These particular aspects correspond to the so-called "dangerous halo" forms, defined by metastases presenting a scalloped appearance at the interface with normal liver tissue. They can be observed in two-stage hepatectomies, and reflect tumor growth occurring after the interruption of induction chemotherapy. The presence of a "dangerous halo" can have an impact on the surgical approach, undermining the possibility of obtaining sufficiently large resection margins and thus increasing the risk of recurrence.

Liver toxicity :

Achieving major regression is the main objective of induction therapy. However, this must be achieved at the cost of reduced toxicity. In this context, the pathologist has a watchdog role in identifying any alterations in liver parenchyma in the vicinity of the metastasis(es). On the one hand, steatohepatitis lesions have been reported after treatment with irinotecan-based chemotherapies, associated with higher postoperative mortality than in patients without such lesions (72). On the other hand, vascular lesions corresponding to sinusoid obstruction syndrome (or SOS syndrome), sometimes associated with nodular regenerative hyperplasia lesions, have been observed after treatment with oxaliplatin (72,73). However, these lesions would be less frequent and severe if this type of chemotherapy were combined with Bevacizumab. This targeted therapy is thought to have a protective effect on the vascular network (73).

Tumor residue:

Must be specified according to Hermanek's classification as (R0, R1 or R2) (74) (table 4).

**Table 4** Hermanek classification.

| | Description |
|---|---|
| R0 | Complete resection, histologically sound margins, no residual tumour left after resection. |
| R1 | Incomplete resection, histologically invaded margins, residual tumour microscopically left after tumour resection. |
| R2 | Incomplete resection, invaded margins or centimetric tumour remnants (macroscopic). |

The extension :

Nodes: The number of nodes removed and the number of metastatic nodes must be specified in the report.

Adventitial nodules: Adventitial nodules or satellite nodules located in the pericolic or perirectal tissue.

Vasculolymphatic emboli: Vasculolymphatic invasion has been considered in numerous studies as an independent prognostic factor in multivariate analysis (75). The prognostic difference between lymphatic and venous invasion has not been established.

Perineural infiltrations: Perineural invasions are less frequent than vasculolymphatic invasions, occurring in 10% of colorectal cancers. They are generally associated with high stage and high grade. The prognostic significance of this criterion has not been demonstrated in all publications. What's more, studies on this subject are few and retrospective (76). The prognostic value of this criterion has therefore not been formally validated for use in clinical practice. (77).
pTNM stage: This must be included at the end of the report, as it is a major prognostic element, the result of several parameters, which primarily conditions the therapeutic attitude.
The pTNM stage corresponds to a histopronostic classification based, after accurate sampling, on the depth of tumor invasion (pT) and its extension into local lymph nodes (pN) and distant lymph nodes (pM), when a metastasis is histologically documented. Survival after diagnosis of colorectal cancer is strongly influenced by histopronostic stage.

Molecular factors :
Colorectal cancers are heterogeneous diseases, and their dismemberment has brought to light molecular alterations and entities with a validated or potential prognostic and/or predictive impact in localized or metastatic situations. These elements are now inseparable from macro- and microscopic elements. They correspond to MSI, BRAF and RAS status.
*Microsatellite instability :*
Colorectal cancers are accompanied by an MSI status (so-called MSI phenotype, or RER for Replication ERror or dMMR for deficient MisMatch Repair, as opposed to the MSS phenotype, stable microsatellite, or pMMR for proficient MisMatch Repair) in 15% of cases. Two-thirds of CRCs with MSI (MSI CRC) occur in a sporadic context, and one-third in a hereditary context (i.e. 2% of all CRCs), as part of Lynch syndrome, formerly known as Hereditary Non Polyposis Colorectal Cancer (HNPCC). The determination of MSI status is based on molecular and/or immunohistochemical tests, which are both equivalent and complementary.
Molecular biology is considered the gold standard, but immunohistochemistry appears to correlate perfectly with it. What's more, immunohistochemistry can be used to identify the altered gene in the event of extinction of a given protein, by exploring the four proteins of the MMR system: hMLH1, hMSH2, hMSH6 and hPMS2. The identification of MSI status is part of the set of prognostic factors for CRC that can guide the therapeutic attitude, and constitutes a screening tool for Lynch syndromes, since it is present in almost all of these hereditary cancers.
Two methods can be used to establish this phenotype:
PCR, by analyzing the amplification products of several regions containing microsatellites and ;
Immunohistochemistry, by studying the expression of proteins encoded by the genes of the MMR (57).
*BRAF gene mutations :*
The BRAF gene codes for the B-Raf protein, a serine/threonine kinase located in the EGFR and MAP kinase pathways. This pathway is deregulated during colorectal carcinogenesis, notably by constitutive activation of BRAF, leading ultimately to

stimulation of cell proliferation and survival. In colorectal cancers, the frequency of BRAF V600E mutation reaches 5-10%, but varies according to certain anatomoclinical features and the molecular group to which the tumor belongs (78). This mutation is more frequent in tumours of proximal location (27%) than in tumours of distal location (3.3%), and occurs more frequently in sporadic MSI CRCs than in MSS CRCs (50-70 and 5-10% respectively). Currently, BRAF mutation testing is mainly used to discriminate between sporadic and hereditary MSI CRCs. These mutations are never found in Lynch syndromes and are observed in 60% of sporadic cases (79). BRAF mutations make it possible to identify patients with a very poor prognosis, particularly in a metastatic context, for whom new therapeutic options need to be defined (80).

*RAS mutations :*

KRAS mutations are associated with resistance to anti-EGFR therapeutic antibodies. The PRIME trial with panitumumab and the FIRE3 trial with cetuximab have demonstrated the major value of a more complete determination of KRAS status, in order to more accurately select patients with metastatic CRC who may benefit from anti-EGFR antibodies (81).

Furthermore, these findings must be made in the context of metastatic disease. The clinical information contained in the report must therefore be as precise as possible, to enable the pathologist to determine the RAS status as quickly as possible. This can also be done as soon as a histologically documented metastasis is examined. The aim of this approach is to reduce the time needed to obtain RAS results, and to optimize the therapeutic strategy for CRC, particularly in first-line metastases.

Summary :

It summarizes the main elements of the report: type of specimen, quality of resection, histological type, grade, histopronostic factors other than pTNM (such as vascular emboli and perineural infiltration), pTNM stage. Its purpose is to provide a summary that can be used immediately in multidisciplinary consultation meetings.

## 7. TNM classification :

### *a) Colon :*

The classification to be used is that proposed by the AJCC and the UICC. It is regularly updated and the latest edition (TNM 8$^{ème}$ edition) has been applicable since 2017.

It is recommended that pathologists specify the classification they use in their reports (Quality Assurance in Pathological Anatomy recommendation).

Examination of at least 12 regional lymph nodes is recommended by the UICC and AJCC to establish TNM N status. Whatever the stage, and particularly for stages II and III, the higher the number of nodes sampled and analyzed, the better the prognosis. The choice of 12 lymph nodes is based on an international consensus (82).

Some studies suggest that the optimal number of nodes to examine depends on the tumor's T status. For stage I tumors, a number of nodes < 12 may be sufficient, and conversely, for T4 tumors, a number of nodes > 12 is more appropriate (83,84).

TNM classification (8ème edition, 2017) :
Tis: intraepithelial or intramucosal carcinoma (carcinoma in situ, intramucosal adenocarcinoma invading the chorion or muscularis mucosa).
T1: tumor invading the submucosa.
T2: tumor invading the muscularis propria.
T3: tumor invading the subserosa.
T4: tumour penetrating the visceral peritoneum and/or invading at least one neighbouring structure/organ.
T4a: penetration of visceral peritoneum*.
T4b: invasion of a neighbouring structure**.

N0: no regional lymph node metastasis.
N1: metastasis in 1 to 3 regional lymph nodes***.
N1a: metastasis in 1 regional lymph node.
N1b: metastases in 2-3 regional lymph nodes.
N1c: "satellite" tumour deposits in the subserosa, or in non-peritonized pericolic or perirectal tissue, in the absence of metastatic lymph node****.
N2: metastasis ≥4 regional lymph nodes.
N2a: metastasis in 4-6 regional lymph nodes.
N2b: metastasis in ≥ 7 regional lymph nodes.
M0: no distant metastases.
M1a: distant metastases confined to an organ without peritoneal involvement: liver, lung, ovary, non-regional lymph nodes, etc.
M1b: metastases reaching more than one metastatic site.
M1c: peritoneal metastasis with or without other organ involvement.

NB: Definition of micro-metastases:
-A tumor focus < 0.2 mm should be classified as N0 ;
-A tumor focus between 0.2 mm and 2 mm in size must be classified as N1 (or higher);
-There is therefore no need to specify pN0 (ITC+) (Isolated Tumor Cells: ITC) or pN1 (MIC) (Micrometastasis: MIC).
* T4a. A T4a stage may correspond to a tumor reaching the surface of the serosa with reactive phenomena (mesothelial hyperplasia, inflammation, erosion or ulceration), to free tumor cells on the surface of the serosa with reactive phenomena of the serosa, or to perforation of the serosa by the tumor with inflammatory reaction.
** T4b A tumor macroscopically adherent to other organs or structures is classified as cT4b. However, if no tumor is microscopically present at the level of adhesion, the histopathological classification will be pT1 to pT3 depending on the depth of infiltration.

*** The regional lymph nodes of the colon are :
- Appendix: ileocolics.
- Cecum: ileocolic, right colic.
- Ascending colon: ileocolic, straight colic, medium colic.
- Right-hepatic angle: medium colic, right colic.
- Transverse colon: right colic, middle colic, left colic, inferior mesenteric.
- Left colic angle: middle colic, left colic, inferior mesenteric.
- Sigmoid colon: sigmoid, left colic, upper rectal, recto-sigmoid and lower mesenteric nodes.

**** : Satellite" tumor deposits correspond to macroscopic or microscopic nodules in peri-colic or peri-rectal adipose tissue, at a distance from the tumor invasion front, with no histological argument in favor of a residual lymph node structure, but in the lymphatic drainage territory of the primary tumor. These deposits may correspond to discontinuous tumour extension, extravascular extension of venous invasion, perivenous infiltration or a completely reworked lymph node, without these structures being identifiable.

In the absence of metastatic lymph nodes, they are classified as N1c. In the presence of metastatic lymph nodes, tumour deposits are reported, but should not be added to metastatic lymph nodes. These definitions are those of the 8ème edition of the TNM classification. They are the subject of debate, with some authors considering that the negative prognostic impact of tumour deposits is not currently sufficiently emphasized (85).

Classification by stage :

| | |
|---|---|
| Stage 0 | pTis N0 M0 |
| Stage I | pT1-2 N0 M0 |
| Stage IIA | pT3 N0 M0 |
| Stage IIB | pT4a N0 M0 |
| Stage IIC | pT4b N0 M0 |
| Stage IIIA | pT1-T2 N1/N1c M0 and pT1 N2a M0 |
| Stage IIIB | pT3-T4a N1N1c M0, pT2-T3 N2a M0, pT1-T2 N2b M0 |
| Stage IIIC | pT4a N2a M0; p T3-T4a N2b M0; pT4b N1-N2 M0 |
| Stage IVA | all T, all N, M1a |
| Stage IVB | all T, all N, M1b |
| IVC stage | all T, all N, M1c |

### *b) Rectum :*

The current classification is that of the UICC (TNM 8th edition 2017).(86).
The regional lymph nodes of the rectum are :
Upper - middle and lower rectal (hemorrhoidal) ganglia (located in the fat of the mesorectum) or mesorectal ganglia (synonymous with rectal ganglion).

Internal iliac (hypogastric) nodes (continuous with the nodes of the middle rectal artery).
Lateral sacral ganglia - presacral and sacral promontory (Gerota) ;
Inferior mesenteric lymph nodes (actually very distant from the rectum and never included in the irradiation fields, but always removed during surgical curage and having a strong prognostic value).
Inguinal nodes in case of anal canal involvement.
Node metastases other than those listed above are classified as distant metastases (obturator or external iliac nodes).
TX Insufficient information to classify the primary tumor.
T0 No evidence of primary tumour.
Tis Carcinoma in situ: intraepithelial or invading the lamina propria.
T1 Tumor invading the submucosa.
T2 Tumor invading the muscularis.
T3 Tumor invading the subserosa or non-peritoneal perirectal tissues.
T4 Tumor directly invading other organs or structures and/or perforating the visceral peritoneum.
T4a Tumor perforating the visceral peritoneum.
T4b Tumor directly invading other organs or structures.
Notes :
1/Tis includes cases of cancer cells confined to the glandular basement membrane (intraepithelial) or lamina propria (intramucosal) without extension through the muscularis mucosa to the submucosa.
2/Direct invasion of a T4b stage includes invasion of other segments of the colon or rectum via the serosal pathway, proven by microscopic examination, or includes, for tumors arising in a retro or subperitoneal location, direct extension to other organs or structures due to extension beyond the mesorectum and fascia recti.
3/A tumor that is macroscopically adherent to other organs or structures is classified as cT4b. However, if there is no tumor cell present in the adherent zone on microscopic examination, it will be classified as pT1-3, depending on the depth of invasion into the wall.

NX Insufficient information to classify regional adenopathies.
N0 No regional lymph node metastasis.
N1 Metastasis in 1 to 3 regional lymph nodes.
N1a Metastases in 1 regional lymph node.
N1b Metastases in 2-3 regional lymph nodes.
N1c Tumour nodule(s), satellite(s)* in the subserosa, or in non-peritonized pericolic or perirectal tissues without regional lymph node metastasis.
N2 Metastasis in ≥ 4 regional lymph nodes.
N2a Metastasis in 4-6 regional lymph nodes.
N2b Metastasis in ≥ 7 regional lymph nodes.

Notes.

*Macroscopic or microscopic tumour nodules (satellites) located in the peri-colic or peri-rectal adipose tissue of the lymphatic drainage zone of the primary tumour, with no histological evidence of residual lymphatic tissue in the nodule, may correspond to discontinuous tumour extension, venous invasion with extravascular extension (V1/2) or a fully tumourized lymph node (N1/2).
If such nodules are observed with tumors that would have been classified as T1 or T2, then the T classification remains unchanged and the nodule is recorded as N1c. If the nodule is considered by the pathologist to be a lymph node totally destroyed by the tumor process (usually of regular contour), it should be recorded as a positive lymph node and not as a satellite nodule, and each should be counted separately to establish the final pN classification.

- M0: no metastasis
- M1: presence of distant metastasis(es)
 M1a Metastasis(es) localized to a single organ (liver, lung, ovary, non-regional lymph node(s)).
 M1b Metastases in more than one organ.
 M1c Metastases in the peritoneum with or without involvement of other organs.
The pT and pN categories correspond to the T and N categories.

The examination of at least 12 regional lymph nodes is necessary to correctly assess lymph node status. If this number is not reached, the specimen must be re-examined by the pathologist. However, in the absence of lymph node involvement, even if the number of 12 nodes usually examined is not reached, TNM 2017, UICC (2002) and AJCC recommend classifying N0 and not Nx patients without node involvement.
Note: the number of lymph nodes is often reduced after neoadjuvant treatment. As a result, the usually required 12 lymph nodes may not be reached despite careful research.
Classification by stage: similar to that for colonic tumours above.
Anatomopathological examination should specify the state of the distal and circumferential margins (clearance) of the resection, as well as the degree of macroscopic integrity of the mesorectum according to Quirke (64). A distal or circumferential margin < 1 mm is considered invaded (R1 resection). A circumferential margin < 2 mm is predictive of local relapse. However, R1 resection is more likely to lead to metastasis than local relapse. In the case of preoperative treatment, the TNM stage on the surgical specimen will be expressed in ypTNM.

# V. Metastatic colorectal cancer:

## A. Diagnosis of MHCCR :

### 1. Positive diagnosis :

#### *a) Circumstances of discovery :*

MH has no specific symptomatology. They should be investigated systematically when CRC is discovered. These MHCCR can be discovered :
-During the initial evaluation of colon or rectal cancer prior to resection, or during manual surgical and/or ultrasound exploration of the liver during resection of the primary tumor. These metastases are said to be synchronous.
-During surveillance after resection of the primary tumor, from a few months to several years. These are known as metachronous tumours.
-Inaugural MH, discovered before the diagnosis of the primary tumor.

#### *b) Clinical manifestations :*

The clinical manifestations of MH are rarely revealing and not very specific. They are mainly observed in advanced forms. The most common functional sign is pain in the right hypochondrium, which is highly suggestive if the patient is a known CRC carrier. Other signs are non-specific, such as minor digestive disturbances, isolated fever or altered general condition.
Occasionally, compression of adjacent structures (main bile duct, portal branch, suprahepatic veins, inferior vena cava) by the metastasis or pedicle adenopathies may determine cholestatic jaundice, portal hypertension or Budd-chiari syndrome.
In addition to these signs, the clinical examination (although usually poor) will look for a typically marooned, firm and tender hepatomegaly with a thrill on palpation or a murmur on auscultation, or a liver with a nodular surface observed in superficial, multiple and/or advanced localizations.

#### *c) Additional tests :*

##### (1) Biological tests :

##### (a) Liver function tests :

The most commonly used blood tests are those for alkaline phosphatase (ALP), transaminase (AST, ALT), bilirubin, gamma glutamyl transferase (GGT) and lactate dehydrogenase (LDH). Biological abnormalities are not very specific or sensitive. They indicate cytolysis and/or cholestasis, with no correlation with MH volume or number. The enzymes with the highest positive predictive value are PAL and GGT.

##### (b) Tumor markers :

Carcinoembryonic antigen (CEA) is the only marker of interest in the management of patients with suspected MHCCR. CEA is more sensitive in detecting hepatic and retroperitoneal lymph node metastases than local, pulmonary or peritoneal recurrences (87).

### (2) Morphological assessment :

#### (a) Transparietal ultrasound (TUS):

FET is the first-line examination, often the first to discover MH. Its specificity for the diagnosis of metastases is excellent, ranging from 85 to 95%. (88)Its sensitivity depends on the size of the lesion: 94% for lesions larger than 2cm and 56% for smaller lesions.

MH lesions most often appear as rounded or polylobed, blurred, echogenic, avascular lesions with a hypoechoic peripheral halo. The center may be fluid in cases of necrosis or mucoid secretion, producing the classic "cockade" appearance. Much more rarely, lesions are anechoic or even hyperechoic.

The advantages of ultrasound - simplicity, safety, low cost, accessibility and reproducibility - make it the first-line examination for screening or assessing secondary liver lesions. However, obesity, steatosis, gastrointestinal gases or a high-situated liver can make the examination difficult, and interpretation depends on the operator.

The use of ultrasound contrast medium further enhances ultrasound performance (89).

Echodoppler may be useful for clarifying the relationships of lesions detected with intrahepatic vessels and the vena cava preoperatively.

#### (b) Computed tomography (CT):

CT is currently the most widely used imaging modality for liver assessment in patients with suspected HD. Helical technology has improved performance, and multiphasic acquisition has enabled better characterization of lesions. In particular, the majority of lesions larger than 1cm are detected by this imaging technique. However, small sub-centimetric lesions are difficult to characterize.

The use of intravenously injected iodinated contrast media is essential for proper exploration of the liver parenchyma. The contrast between liver lesions and the rest of the liver parenchyma will depend on the total dose injected, the injection rate and the acquisition time.

Metastases appear as nodular or polycyclic lesions, iso or hypodense, with early and transient peripheral contrast after intravenous injection of contrast medium. Lesions may sometimes be hyperdense in cases of hemorrhage or calcification.

The sensitivity of CT scans for the detection of CBMs is between 75 and 85%, while specificity remains good, at between 85 and 97%.

Portal slices are the most effective for detecting hepatic lesions. To better characterize the lesions detected, acquisitions are made at different vascular times (arterial time, portal time, late time) and/or further exploration by directed ultrasound is recommended. In this way, the liver lesion can be clearly delimited, and its relationship with vascular structures clarified. It can also be used to assess the resectability of the lesion, by measuring the remaining liver volume if a wide resection is planned.

#### (c) Magnetic resonance imaging MRI :

Hepatic MRI with contrast injection is the most sensitive preoperative examination for detecting and characterizing secondary hepatic lesions.

This is a non-irradiating technique, and the contrast agents used have low nephrotoxicity and are less allergenic than iodinated contrast agents. Recently, three-dimensional acquisitions have made it possible to perform true volume mapping of the liver and vessels.

MRI with or without gadolinium injection is no better than helical CT for detecting liver metastases, with sensitivity ranging from 66% to 83%. It is indicated when CT is not possible (high risks associated with the use of iodinated PC: allergy, renal insufficiency), or when CT is insufficient to characterize the liver lesions detected. It is also of interest in cases of hepatic steatosis.

### (d) Positron emission tomography (PET) :

PET differs from other functional imaging methods in that it is based on the general principle of scintigraphy, which involves injecting photon-emitting radioactive tracers (67 gallium, 201 thallium, MTC MIBI), the most widely used recently being [F-8]-Fluoro-2-deoxyglucose (FDG).

Sensitivity and specificity are 88% and 96% respectively for PET. PET is therefore a powerful tool for the assessment of MHCCR, as well as for extrahepatic lesions. It is also useful for detecting local recurrence of the primary tumor. PET is showing increasing promise for follow-up after radiofrequency treatment of HCM.

However, although PET appears to be a high-performance diagnostic imaging tool for MHCCR, it is not routinely used, due to its cost and limited availability.

### (e) Intraoperative ultrasound :

It provides the surgeon with additional information on the internal structure of the liver, unknown to other morphological explorations, enabling perfect identification of the vascular and biliary relationships of metastases.

Its sensitivity (95-99%) and specificity (95-100%) are significantly higher than those of preoperative ultrasound.

### (f) Others :

#### *(i) Percutaneous ultrasound-guided liver biopsy:*

Histological confirmation is only indicated if the metastasis is discovered before the primary tumor, or when the context and/or imaging - in particular MRI with gadolinium injection - are not sufficient to characterize a hepatic lesion. However, liver biopsy in a neoplastic context requires special precautions: use coaxial needles, avoid repeated punctures and biopsy subcapsular tumors without interposition of healthy parenchyma. Although the risk of tumour dissemination along the puncture route is minimal (<1%), it is worth noting.

#### *(ii) Radioimmunodetection :*

Its principle is to direct a gamma-emitting isotope at tumor cells using a monoclonal antibody directed against a tumor antigen.

The results for MH are disappointing: although specificity is often over 90%, sensitivity is low, at around 50-70%.

## 2. Differential diagnosis :

It can be performed in cases of synchronous MH or if the primary cancer is unknown.

### *a) Biliary cysts :*

These are the most common liver malformations. They are fluid-filled cavities lined with biliary epithelium. They are easily recognized by their ultrasound appearance: spherical or oval image, sharp margins, anechogenic with posterior enhancement.

### *b) Angiomas or hemangiomas :*

They are also frequent and appear hyperechoic on ultrasound. This poses a problem of differential diagnosis with hyperechoic MH, which is why a CT scan with injection of contrast medium, or even an MRI, is necessary.

### *c) Liver abscess :*

Whose ultrasound appearance (anechoic center) associated with fever may lead to confusion with MH necrosis.

### *d) Hydatid cyst of the liver:*

In its pseudotumor or calcified form.

### *e) Other malignant liver tumors :*

Hepatocellular carcinoma, cholangiocarcinoma, neuroendocrine metastases.

### *f) Other benign tumors :*

Focal nodular hyperplasia, adenoma, cystadenoma, polycystic liver disease.

## B. Pre-therapeutic assessment :

Once the diagnosis of MHCCR has been made, the choice of treatment depends on the extent of the disease and the patient's operability.

## 1. Assessment of extension :

Complete surgical resection is the only curative treatment for MHCCR. For this reason, it is essential to rely on an optimal workup that detects all intra- and extra-hepatic tumor disease.

### *a) Liver disease:*

Helical CT, MRI and PET scans are now considered to be the most effective.
CT scans, possibly with three-dimensional reconstructions, or MRI with frontal slices, can be used to determine the extent and location of metastases in relation to biliary structures, and portal and supra-hepatic vessels, which are decisive factors in resectability.
MRI with injection of liver-specific contrast medium (Ferumoxide) is the most sensitive preoperative examination for the detection of CBM.
Predictive assessment of the remaining liver volume, based on CT or MRI images, is recommended for large resections.

### *b) Extrahepatic disease:*

Discussion of the resectability of MHCCR requires a complete workup of the disease:

-Clinical examination must be thorough, looking for signs of extra-hepatic metastases: abdominal examination and rectal examination, looking for peritoneal carcinosis, palpation of lymph nodes in search of a Troisier node.
-Morphological examinations should include at least a thoraco-abdomino-pelvic CT scan to look for pulmonary or intra-abdominal metastases (ovaries, adrenals). X-rays, CT scans and scintigraphy are the examinations of choice for bone metastases, which are essential in the presence of bone pain or pathological fractures. Finally, PET scans may be considered, as they appear to be effective in assessing extrahepatic disease.
The CEA level measured at the time of the extension work-up does not modify the therapeutic attitude, but its measurement is useful for monitoring the response to treatment.

## 2. **Operability report :**

This check-up is essential, as it is before any type of surgery. It includes an assessment of the patient's general condition, an anaesthesia consultation, complementary examinations based on the results of the clinical examination and the planned surgery (laparoscopy, resection, clamping), and transfusion requirements.
In addition to the usual complementary tests (chest X-ray, ECG, blood grouping, CBC, ionogram, blood cell count, etc.), specific liver tests (albuminemia, bilirubinemia, serum PAL, GGT, transaminases, prothrombin level) are also performed.
Other tests have been proposed to assess non-tumoral liver function, such as hepatic clearance studies, loading tests (e.g. with glucose) or scintigraphy, the indocyanine green retention test, a dye eliminated exclusively by the liver. This is a true liver function test, enabling assessment of hepatic blood flow. Retention after 15 minutes is normally less than 10%; retention of more than 30% contraindicates liver resection.
Assessment of the patient's nutritional status is mandatory prior to hepatectomy, especially if the operation is to be major or associated with colorectal resection. If the patient's general condition deteriorates, attempts should be made to improve it by continuous enteral or parenteral nutrition. The timing of hepatectomy should be reconsidered, at least initially, until the patient's nutritional status improves.
Preoperative assessment of respiratory function is important, given the impact of liver surgery, pneumoperitoneum, diaphragmatic paralysis and impaired ventilatory mechanics. Assessment of the heart's condition is also vital, in order to evaluate the cardiac tolerance to different types of clamping.
In fact, the anaesthetic work-up is not really specific, and only the physiological age counts. However, it is important to discuss with the anaesthetist the particularities of the surgery, which may, for example, require hepatic pedicle clamping or even vascular exclusion, and to carefully assess the risk/benefit ratio, all the more so if the patient is elderly or at high anaesthetic risk.
A possible contraindication to laparoscopy must be systematically sought.

### C. Pre-therapeutic classification :

Pre-therapeutic classification helps guide the management strategy:
1. TNM c classification :
2. For rectal cancers: Topography (low, medium or high), CRM.
3. MH resectable type I and II.
4. ASA classification, WHO.
5. Molecular classification: RAS, BRAF, MSI.

### D. Treatment strategy :

The last two decades have seen considerable upheaval in the therapeutic armamentarium and strategy for metastatic CRC, with the advent of more active cytotoxic anticancer agents (oxaliplatin, irinotecan) on the one hand, agents targeting tumor angiogenesis or the epidermal growth factor receptor (EGFR) on the other, and advances in the medical-surgical management of metastases (90).
Approximately 20% of patients with CRC have HSM at diagnosis. If liver lesions are deemed resectable after a thorough preoperative work-up, only surgical treatment of the colorectal tumour and liver lesions will be associated with prolonged survival. However, for patients with unresectable metastases, the management strategy aims to improve quality of life or, at best, achieve a high rate of conversion to resectable status, which alone opens the door to curative treatment and prolonged survival. In addition to the management of liver metastases and methods to increase their resectability rate, the synchronous nature of the disease poses the problem of the management of the primary colonic or rectal tumour, and above all the chronology of its management in relation to the surgery of the metastases. (91).
Treatment of liver metastases must be tailored to the characteristics and objectives of each individual patient.
Patients with liver metastases of colorectal origin can be classified into three groups:
**Group 1: readily resectable metastases:** Nordlinger's Phase III trial showed that pre- and post-operative chemotherapy with FOLFOX reduced the risk of cancer recurrence (92,93). Small metastases that might disappear under chemotherapy and pose problems for intra-operative location can be removed from the outset.
-**Group 2: Potentially resectable metastases:** Metastases are not immediately surgically resectable, but may become so in the event of significant regression during chemotherapy. Patients must be able to withstand aggressive chemotherapy. In such cases, chemotherapies that produce a significant and rapid response are preferred (94). When the RAS gene is mutated, chemotherapy is combined with an antiangiogenic agent, notably Bevacizumab. When the RAS gene is not mutated, three clinical trials showed no major difference between cytotoxics combined with Bevacizumab, and cytotoxics combined with anti-EGFR, Cetuximab, or Panitumumab (95).
It is very important that these patients are regularly reassessed at a multidisciplinary consultation meeting, so that chemotherapy can be suspended as soon as the metastases become resectable, and to avoid prolonging

chemotherapy unnecessarily, which could induce damage to the liver parenchyma that could prohibit any subsequent surgery.
The aim of surgery is to achieve complete removal (R0) of liver metastases with low operative morbidity and mortality.
Complete surgical excision is the curative treatment for liver metastases of colorectal origin. The volume of liver remaining after excision should be at least 30-40% of the initial total volume (96).
**-Group 3**: **Disseminated metastases:** These are unlikely to become accessible to surgery. The aim of drug treatment is not curative.
Combinations of Fluoro-pyrimide and Oxaliplatin (FOLFOX) or Irinotecan (FOLFIRI) coupled with targeted therapy are generally used.
The combination of Fluoro-pyrimidines (5FU or Capecitabine) with Bevacizumab in elderly patients (>70 years) is well tolerated with better oncological results than Capecitabine alone (AVEX trial) (97) .
This raises questions about treatment duration, dose reduction to improve tolerance, and therapeutic pauses to enhance patient comfort. In patients in good clinical condition, it is essential to maintain the principle of reassessment during PCR, because even in this group, unexpected responses to chemotherapy may lead to reconsideration of the possibility of surgical excision.
When metastases are disseminated and symptomatic, the aim is to prevent tumor progression and improve symptoms with a well-tolerated treatment.
The therapeutic strategy is defined in agreement with the patient, based on the advice of the multidisciplinary consultation meeting (RCP).

Synchronous liver metastases:
The international multidisciplinary consensus on the management of synchronous liver metastases from colorectal cancer (98) distinguishes three groups of liver metastases with different prognoses, depending on the time of diagnosis:
1-Synchronous liver metastases: which should be referred to as "synchronously detected liver metastases", these are defined as any liver metastases detected at or before the diagnosis of the primary tumor.
2-Early metachronous metastases: these are metastases detected within 12 months of diagnosis or surgery of the primary tumour.
3-Late metachronous metastases: these are metastases detected more than 12 months after diagnosis or surgery of the primary tumour.

**Asymptomatic colorectal cancer and resectable synchronous HD**: Surgery for liver metastases is accompanied by perioperative chemotherapy.
Combined surgery is indicated for patients with limited liver disease and an easily resectable primary tumor.

**Asymptomatic colorectal cancer and unresectable synchronous MH ˝d'emblée˝ :**

Traditionally, the primary tumour was resected first, followed by chemotherapy and then resection of liver metastases when resectability was achieved. Today,

chemotherapy combined with targeted therapy is administered first, with the aim of rendering liver metastases resectable.
If MH becomes resectable, reverse surgery (liver first) is recommended.

**Symptomatic colorectal cancer and resectable synchronous HD:**
Colorectal cancer can be symptomatic, causing haemorrhage, obstruction or perforation. The primary tumor should be resected first, followed by chemotherapy and then surgery for the MH.

**Symptomatic colorectal cancer and synchronous unresectable MH ˝d'emblée˝ :**
Resection of the primary tumor, followed by chemotherapy, then surgery for HD if it becomes resectable.

At least four courses of optimal first-line chemotherapy (bichimiotherapy with targeted therapy or trichimiotherapy with targeted therapy) are recommended for potentially resectable metastases, with response assessment every 2 months and a total duration (preoperative and adjuvant) of 6 months of systemic treatment.

**Special features of metastatic rectal cancer** (99):

Management of rectal cancers with resectable synchronous liver metastases:
In the case of rectal cancer with resectable MH, curative treatment should be considered. In the case of the rectum, treatment is based on excision of the tumour from the rectum and mesorectum with healthy surgical margins, more or less preceded by radio-chemotherapy (RCT). In the case of resectable MH, treatment is based on complete excision surgery accompanied by perioperative oxaliplatin-based chemotherapy (92). Synchronous presentation of metastatic disease and its optimal treatment must not compromise optimal treatment of rectal cancer, and vice versa. The therapeutic strategy will therefore depend on the location and extent of the rectal tumour, the extent of the metastatic disease, the surgical procedure envisaged on the liver and the patient's general condition. Broadly speaking, defining the therapeutic strategy in this complex clinical situation comes down to answering 2 questions:
-Should the presence of synchronous MH lead to changes in the preoperative treatment of rectal cancer?
-When should synchronous HD be operated on? Should it be operated on at the same time as rectal cancer, or separately from rectal cancer?
In the latter case, should the MH be operated on after (classic approach) or before (reverse approach) rectal cancer?

Should preoperative treatment of rectal cancer be modified in the case of synchronous liver metastases?
No study has evaluated the value of preoperative treatments, i.e. radiotherapy or RCT, in rectal cancer with resectable synchronous HD. The most scientifically robust data available are from controlled trials on the management of patients with non-metastatic rectal cancer:

For cancers of the middle or lower rectum T1-T2 N0 or for metastatic tumors of the upper rectum, by analogy with a non-metastatic situation, there is a priori no indication for preoperative treatment. (100).
In this situation, the only question will be when to operate on MH in relation to rectal cancer.
-For locally advanced tumors of the middle or lower rectum (T3/T4 and/or N+) that are not immediately R0 resectable, i.e. with a predictable circumferential margin on MRI of less than 1 mm. In this situation, treatment will depend on the extent of metastatic disease.
In the case of locally advanced unresectable R0 rectal cancer with minimal MH, tumor reduction is necessary before considering R0 rectal excision surgery. In this situation, short 5x5 Gy radiotherapy over one week is not appropriate. Preoperative CTR helps to achieve tumor regression and limit the risk of local recurrence after rectal excision surgery (100). In this situation, the main disadvantage of RCT is the progression of small, resectable MH that becomes unresectable during treatment. This theoretical risk has been little evaluated, but could be real insofar as the type of regimen and dose of chemotherapy administered to potentiate the effect of irradiation may be considered suboptimal for treating metastatic disease.
A bicentric study conducted at Ambroise Paré and Bicêtre hospitals assessed the fate of 41 MHs undergoing RCT in 20 patients with locally advanced rectal cancer with resectable synchronous MHs (101).
In this study, a lesion-by-lesion analysis of MH response was carried out and showed that the majority of MHs (83%) were stable during RCT.
In the case of locally advanced unresectable R0 rectal cancer with extensive MH, the same strategy could be discussed, but given the extension of metastatic disease, the risk of initially resectable MH becoming unresectable is greater. This is why, in this situation, initial chemotherapy may be an alternative to RCT, as it provides more reliable control of the metastatic disease and, depending on the response, offers the possibility of starting with surgery for HD.
In the case of R0 resectable T3 or N+ cancer, i.e. with MRC > 1 mm on MRI, here again the strategy will depend on metastatic extension, and numerous options are possible. Indeed, in this situation where rectal cancer can be resected R0, the value of preoperative treatment whose sole aim is to reduce the risk of local recurrence is more debatable, given the presence of CBM. If the MH is not very extensive, we can propose surgery from the outset, short radiotherapy or RCT, whereas in the case of extensive MH, we tend to propose chemotherapy alone.

When to operate on liver metastases synchronous with rectal cancer?
The first question is whether it is preferable to resect HD at the same time or separately from rectal surgery. Simultaneous resection of rectal cancer and synchronous HD is feasible with low morbidity and mortality in selected patients and in trained teams. Laparoscopic rectal resection could facilitate the post-operative management of this combined approach. (18). On the other hand, simultaneous resection is contraindicated in cases of intraoperative discovery of MH, emergency surgery for rectal cancer, and complex liver or rectal surgery. A

combined approach should always be discussed at the RCP in the case of bilateral resectable MH for which a 2-stage hepatic resection is envisaged, in order to couple the rectal resection with the simplest first stage of hepatic resection (102). However, in this situation, the first stage of hepatic resection coupled with rectal resection must be limited to metastasectomy or radiofrequency, as it has been reported that in the event of complication of this combined surgery, the 2ème stage of hepatic resection is practically never performed. (103). More than 20 retrospective studies and one meta-analysis (14) compared these two approaches (combined or sequential) and, with one exception (20)concluded that there was no difference in immediate operative or mid-term oncological outcomes. None of these studies was specifically devoted to rectal cancer, and the number of patients included who had rectal cancer was usually less than 60. All these studies are difficult to interpret, since patients who had one or other of these attitudes were not comparable. Indeed, the majority of patients with a rectal primary were included in the separate excision group, as were patients with the most extensive MH. Currently, in the absence of robust data in the literature, separate resection of rectal cancer and resectable HD remains the rule in the majority of cases.
In the case of separate resections, two approaches are possible: the "classic" sequence, involving initial removal of the rectal tumour followed by surgery of the MH, and a reversed approach involving initial removal of the MH followed by removal of the rectal primary in a second operation. The advantages of the "classic" sequence are that it avoids the risk of progression and complications of the primary tumor, and therefore facilitates the administration of treatments targeting metastatic disease. The main drawback of this approach is the risk of progression of metastatic disease, which becomes inaccessible to curative excision during treatment of the primary tumor. This risk may be further increased by postoperative morbidity after rectal excision, delaying treatment of the metastatic disease.
Advances in chemotherapy over the past two decades have led to the development of the reverse strategy concept. This approach was initially proposed for the management of patients with initially unresectable MH who had responded well to chemotherapy (11).
The advantages of this reverse strategy are to enable immediate and optimal control of the metastatic disease, particularly in the case of advanced metastatic disease, and to enable appropriate treatment of the primary tumor, including, if necessary, preoperative treatment when the metastatic disease has been treated. The main drawback of this strategy is the risk of complications linked to the primary tumor during chemotherapy and during removal of the MH.
Few studies have compared the feasibility, postoperative and oncological outcomes of these different approaches.
Two recent retrospective studies have shown that the postoperative results of the different approaches were similar in terms of morbidity in selected patients (104).

Summary and proposed treatment :
In summary, the management of patients with resectable rectal cancer must be defined as curative. Although the prognosis depends primarily on the metastatic

course of the disease, this management must ensure optimal treatment not only of the metastatic disease, but also of the rectal cancer, avoiding incomplete resection at all costs (R1). The appropriate use of preoperative treatment according to local extension, including in patients with synchronous MH, should be the rule, and should help limit the risk of local recurrence. In other words, optimal treatment of one tumour site must not compromise optimal treatment of the other.

For practical use

In the case of small rectal cancers with extensive MH, the treatment strategy begins with chemotherapy, followed by a reverse strategy involving surgery of the MH first, followed by surgery of the rectum +/- preceded by short radiotherapy or RCT.

This approach seems to us to be the most appropriate, as it ensures that the window of resectability of HD is not missed, and in this situation, the value of preoperative treatment of rectal cancer is debatable.

In the case of a large rectal cancer in the presence of a small amount of CBM, the strategy begins with RCT, followed by a conventional strategy involving primary surgery of the rectal cancer, followed by removal of the CBM +/- preceded by chemotherapy. The first RCT will ensure tumour reduction, enabling R0 removal of the rectal tumour.

In the case of large rectal cancers with extensive HD, the strategy starts with chemotherapy, then a reverse strategy may be proposed if the rectal tumor is not obstructive and has responded well to chemotherapy.

In this case, the strategy is first to perform surgery on the MH, followed by surgery on the rectum, preceded by RCT. This is, of course, the most serious situation.

The attitude is to first treat the metastatic disease that dominates the oncological prognosis. However, it is in this situation that the risk of incomplete or inappropriate treatment of rectal cancer is greatest. In these patients, preoperative treatment of rectal cancer based on RCT is essential to avoid R1 excisions in patients who have otherwise been treated for advanced metastatic disease.

In the case of small rectal cancers with a small amount of MH, anything is possible, and in theory, these patients have the best prognosis. No precise recommendation can be made, apart from the need to administer preoperative chemotherapy before excision of HD. It is possible to propose chemotherapy followed by simultaneous surgery, or RCT followed by rectal surgery +/- combined with CBM removal, or short 25 Gy radiotherapy followed by rectal surgery followed by chemo and CBM removal. (99).

## E. Processing :

In recent years, considerable progress has been made in the treatment of patients with MHCCR. Therapeutic means such as surgery, chemotherapy and local destruction methods have improved.

Multidisciplinary management has become a guarantee of treatment quality.

1. **Surgical resection:**

## *a) Vis-à-vis colorectal cancer :*

Laparoscopic or laparotomy colorectal resection is performed in compliance with carcinological rules, with proximal vessel ligation, lymph node curage, and respect for distal, proximal and circumferential margins.
Several types of resection are described, depending on the topography and extent of excision:
Right hemicolectomy, left hemicolectomy, left high segmental resection, left low segmental resection, anterior resection with partial or total exeresis of the mesorectum, abdominoperineal amputation, Hartmann procedure...
Continuity is re-established by mechanical or manual anastomosis, depending on tumour location. The anastomosis is protected by a lateral ileostomy in the case of subperitoneal anastomosis.
A left iliac colostomy is performed in cases of abdominoperineal amputation or Hartmann surgery.

## *b) Vis-à-vis liver metastases:*

Until now, surgical excision of liver metastases has been the only curative treatment option to achieve significantly better medium- and long-term survival rates than other treatments.
Resection of liver metastases from colorectal cancer is effective, with 5-year survival rates ranging from 35% to 58%, whereas 5-year survival is virtually nil in the absence of resection. (7).
Hepatic resection is currently performed with low morbidity and an operative mortality of around 1% in specialized centers. However, only 10-20% of patients with liver metastases from colorectal cancer are eligible for resection.

### (1) Classification of hepatectomies :

Hepatic resection techniques encompass all procedures aimed at resecting one or more of the eight segments of the liver.

#### (a) Typical and atypical hepatectomies:

Hepatectomies can be divided into three main groups:
-Typical (anatomical) hepatectomies are defined by an exeresis limited by an anatomical scissure plane: we therefore speak of right or left hepatectomy (hemihepatectomy), sectoriectomy or segmentectomy;
Atypical (non-anatomical) hepatectomies consist of an excision which does not correspond to an anatomical part of the liver and therefore whose plane of section does not pass through an anatomical scissure;

-Lumpectomies or metastasectomies remove only the tumour, with a safety margin of liver parenchyma.
The term "regulated hepatectomy" refers to hepatectomies with primary vascular control. It is contrasted with parenchymal hepatectomies without vascular control. Typical hepatectomies can therefore be "regulated" or not, and vice versa. It seems easier to speak of anatomical hepatectomy (or not) with (or without) primary vascular control, specifying the level of this vascular control: isolated portal or portal and suprahepatic or portal, suprahepatic and inferior vena cava.

### *(i) Anatomical designation of hepatectomies (105) According to Brisbane nomenclature.*

Anatomical hepatectomies are named according to the contiguous liver segments they remove.
Right hepatectomy (four segments) and left hepatectomy (three segments) are referred to as "major" hepatectomies. Trisegmentectomies, in particular the more common 6, 5 and 4 and the central trisegmentectomy 8, 5 and 4 or 5,4 and 1, are assimilated to major hepatectomies.
Hepatectomies that remove more segments than a major hepatectomy are called "extended". These are right hepatectomy enlarged to segment 4 or segment 1 (removing five segments) and left hepatectomy enlarged to segment 1 (four segments). Super-expanded hepatectomy" is defined as a right hepatectomy enlarged to segments 4 and 1, or a left hepatectomy enlarged to segments 8, 5 and 1 (six segments), or a left hepatectomy enlarged to segments 8 and 5 (five segments).
Other anatomical hepatectomies are limited hepatectomies whose name depends on the segments removed:
- Segmentectomies: removal of a single segment (named after the segment removed).
- Bisegmentectomy: removal of 2 segments.
- Trisegmentectomy: removal of 3 segments.
- Left hepatectomy: removal of segments 2, 3 and 4.
- Right hepatectomy: removal of segments 5, 6, 7, 8.
- Left lobectomy: removal of segments 2 and 3.
- Right lobectomy: removal of segments 4, 5, 6, 7 and 8.

### *(ii) Rules to follow :*

Whatever the type of resection chosen, a number of rules must be observed to avoid postoperative complications.
-Preservation of functional parenchyma corresponding to at least 30 to 40% of liver mass to avoid the risk of postoperative liver failure (96).
-Limitation of intraoperative blood loss in order to reduce the need for blood transfusion, which has been shown to be a factor favoring recurrence and postoperative morbidity and mortality (106,107).
-A safety margin of at least 1 cm must be maintained to reduce the risk of recurrence and avoid compromising the expected survival benefit.

-Respect the glissonian pedicles destined for the remaining segments, so as not to leave an excluded or poorly vascularized sector, a source of ischemia and necrosis as well as biliary fistula.

### (b) Resectability criteria

Two assumptions have already been made:

-Complete surgical resection of hepatic metastases from colorectal cancer (MHCCR) remains the only treatment that leads to a cure.

-Partial resection, which leaves tumor tissue in place, is to be avoided, as it has no therapeutic value.

Liver resection should therefore only be undertaken if its completeness is foreseeable. However, partial resection can sometimes be part of a surgical strategy involving a two-stage hepatectomy.

The resectability of MHCCR must be discussed systematically on the basis of technical and carcinological criteria, during a multidisciplinary medical-surgical consultation within a multidisciplinary oncology consultation meeting (RCP), including a surgeon and a radiologist experienced in liver pathology.

A metastasis is defined as resectable if a hepatectomy can be performed to remove all tumour tissue (R0 resection) with an acceptable operative risk.

### (c) Technical evaluation of resectability :

#### *(i) Methods :*

The evaluation of the resectability of MHCCR includes:

Optimum preoperative assessment: the detection of all intra- and extra-hepatic tumour mass, as well as the vascular relationships of the hepatic tumour(s), are the determining factors in resectability.

-As complete an intraoperative assessment as possible: systematic visual and palpatory exploration of the liver and abdominal cavity, and intraoperative ultrasound for final assessment of resectability.

Laparoscopic exploration with echolaparoscopy can be proposed as part of the resectability assessment, particularly in cases of strong preoperative suspicion of irresectability (suspected carcinosis), thus avoiding unnecessary laparotomies.

#### (a) Technical" definition of resectability:

One or more MHCCRs are technically resectable if:

-Hepatectomy leaves the parenchyma intact, with its own vascularization and biliary drainage (anatomical feasibility),

-The remaining parenchyma is sufficient to ensure satisfactory hepatocellular function (volumetric and functional assessment),

-Predicted operative mortality and morbidity are minimal.

#### *(i) Assessment of anatomical feasibility of resection :*

In the case of single or multiple unilobar tumors, technical contraindications are exceptional. In the case of bilateral multiple tumors :

-The number and location of metastases may be a factor in unresectability. Total hepatectomy to eradicate all lesions with transplantation is not an option.

-The vascular relationships of the various tumors are often the limiting factor: involvement of both right and left portal pedicles, invasion of a portal pedicle by a metastasis and of the contralateral suprahepatic vein(s) by another lesion, or even partial involvement of all three suprahepatic veins.
Management of these vascular problems may involve complex hepatectomy techniques with vascular reconstruction, which can only be performed and evaluated in selected cases within a specialized team.

#### *(ii) Volumetric and functional evaluation :*

Functional assessment of the remaining parenchyma must be both quantitative (validated volumetric calculation based on CT scan) and qualitative, bearing in mind that estimates of this residual tolerable volume in the literature range from 30% to 40%. (96).
Today, reliable and validated means are available to perform this calculation. Volumes are extrapolated from CT images, and advances in imaging technology have improved the accuracy of these calculations (fast-acquisition CT, three-dimensional reconstructions, integrated software).

#### *(iii) Surgical risk assessment :*

The anesthetic evaluation must take into account the planned procedure and the clamping method. Age in itself should not be a contraindication to hepatectomy; only physiological age should be taken into account.
Surgical technique (extent of resection, clamping, vascular control) must be designed to prevent the main risks of hepatectomy: hemorrhage, hemodynamic disturbances, gas embolism and hepatocellular failure. Technical resectability in the case of re-hepatectomies must be based on the same anatomical and volumetric reasoning as for the first hepatectomy.

### (b) Carcinological criteria for resectability :

The decision to resect MHCCR from the outset must take into account all the carcinological features of the disease.

#### *(i) Factors dependent on the initial disease :*

In the case of synchronous metastases, hepatic resection can be performed at the same time as the primary tumour resection (combined resection) if the appropriate skills are available. Combined resection is therefore left to the surgeon's discretion, but is not recommended in the following circumstances: emergency colon surgery, locally advanced colorectal disease or liver disease requiring major resection.

#### *(ii) Factors related to liver disease :*

In cases of Class I resectability, none of the following criteria, even if individually recognized as poor prognostic factors, should limit the indication for surgery: size, number, bilobar character of RCMs, vascular or biliary invasion, CEA levels.
On the other hand, in cases of Class II resectability, preoperative chemotherapy is required.
A re-hepatectomy is justified on the same criteria as for the first hepatectomy.

### *(iii) Factors related to surgical technique :*

The margin of safety: The existence of an invaded margin is recognized as equivalent to palliative intervention. The need for R0 intervention is therefore recognized and agreed upon. Regarding the required thickness of this margin of safety, determining a precise "mandatory" value is difficult, and illusory. Studies have suggested that the resection margin should be at least 1cm to ensure a 5-year survival rate of around 45%. Ambiru et al. (108) studying resection specimens from 168 resected patients, found micrometastases in 31% of cases, located at an average distance of 3mm, while Kokudo et al. (109) stated that a 2mm resection margin was sufficient in the majority of cases.
It is recommended to have a provisional margin of 1cm, and at least 5 mm (expert agreement). (110) .

Type of excision: There is no argument for recommending atypical or anatomical excision when the choice between the two procedures is possible, as the margin factor is paramount in this respect.

### *(iv) Factors dependent on extrahepatic disease :*

-Pedicle or celiac lymph node involvement:
A definite preoperative diagnosis of locoregional metastatic adenopathy(ies) is a contraindication to immediate surgery. A visual and palpatory examination of the pedicle and celiac lymph nodes must be carried out prior to any hepatic procedure; any suspicious lymph node (by its size or texture) must be removed for extemporaneous examination.
In the case of an invaded pedicle node, if resectability is class I, surgery with curage cannot be contraindicated, but this decision must nevertheless be part of a multidisciplinary approach. On the other hand, if resectability is class II, surgery is not recommended.

-Other intra-abdominal locations :
An extrahepatic tumor site that is not completely resectable (non-R0) is a contraindication to hepatectomy.
If this extrahepatic location is resectable: hepatectomy combined with resection of extrahepatic disease or contact invasion is feasible from the outset. Nevertheless, the existence of several pejorative carcinological features of the liver disease and/or the need to perform a class II hepatectomy prompt discussion of initial chemotherapy.

-Extra-abdominal metastatic disease :
The existence of unresectable pulmonary metastasis(es) or extra-abdominal non-lung localization(s) (bone, brain, extra-abdominal adenopathies) contraindicates liver resection.
The discovery of resectable pulmonary metastasis(es) should prompt us to verify the isolated nature of both locations and, in this case, consider double curative surgery. Liver surgery should be performed first.

### (d) Surgical technique :

### *(i) Installation:*

Patient positioning is the same for all abdominal incisions. The patient is positioned supine, with arms crossed at the anaesthetic team's disposal, or with the right arm alongside the body. A suitable log (rolled sheets, or ideally a gel log) is placed under the patient, at the point of the shoulder blades, allowing better exposure, particularly of the celiac region. Some surgeons prefer to place the log under the right hemi-abdomen to facilitate exposure of the posterior aspect of the right liver and the right edge of the inferior vena cava.

### *(ii) Approach :*

-A right bi-subcostal incision: This is made approximately 5 cm below the costal margin. A median split line can be added to provide better access to the upper segments of the liver (segments IVa, VII, VIII).

-Midline incision: A midline incision can be used to perform a hepatectomy, even on the right liver. The advantage of this incision is that it is simpler to perform and close, and therefore likely to reduce operative time. However, median incisions are known to be more painful, with greater pulmonary impact.

-The Makuuchi or J incision: is a median incision starting below the xiphoid, extending up to 5 cm above the umbilicus, before obliquing in a "J" towards the ninth intercostal space, down to the posterior axillary line. Exposure is then achieved by folding up the musculocutaneous flap, which is held in place by valves attached to each of the posts.

-Modified Makuuchi incision: Recently, Vauthey proposed a modified Maakuchi incision (111). The midline incision is continued to the umbilicus, then obliquely perpendicular in the right flank, in an "L" shape. The theoretical advantages of this incision would be that the horizontal branch would be parallel to the metameric distribution of the dermatomes, thus preserving the vascularization and innervation of the wall.

-Laparoscopy: Although initial experience was mainly with benign lesions, resections for malignant tumors (hepatic metastases, hepatocellular carcinoma) are now being performed. Early experience shows the feasibility and safety of laparoscopic resection in patients selected on the basis of the favorable size and topography of their lesions (anterior and lateral segments, size<5cm, at a distance from the hilum and vena cava). Most often, these are limited resections (<3 segments), but major hepatectomies are also feasible. Left lobectomy is the most reproducible of all laparoscopic liver resections. The advantages are those of any laparoscopic procedure (parietal preservation and earlier return to previous activities).

This approach is now possible, but requires mastery of laparoscopic and liver surgery techniques.

### *(iii) Abdominal exploration :*

At the submesocolic level, the entire small bowel is unrolled to look for carcinomatous nodules. The mesos and medial retroperitoneum are also inspected for metastatic adenopathy or nodules of carcinosis.

In the supramesocolic region, adenopathies of the hepatic pedicle, duodeno-pancreatic region and celiac trunk are sought. The diaphragmatic cupolas are thoroughly explored.
In the liver parenchyma, an initial assessment of the number, location and size of metastases is made by palpation. Suspected lesions are biopsied for extemporaneous anatomopathological examination. When the liver parenchyma does not appear macroscopically healthy, or when a major hepatectomy is envisaged (≥ three segments), a biopsy of the non-tumoral liver is taken for extemporaneous examination to assess the quality of the liver parenchyma (steatosis, fibrosis, cirrhosis).

### *(iv) Preparing the liver :*

The round ligament is sectioned and kept long. The falciform, right and left triangular ligaments are also sectioned. With the liver fully mobilized, intraoperative ultrasound can be performed under excellent conditions.

### *(v) Intraoperative ultrasound :*

It enables the discovery of lesions that cannot be palpated, and confirms lesions that have already been palpated or visualized by specifying their size. In addition, this examination clarifies the relationship of metastases to glissonian pedicles and suprahepatic veins, enabling us to determine the planes of parenchymal section that are marked on the surface of the liver.

### *(vi) Vascular control :*

At the level of the hepatic pedicle, a variation in the arterial vascularization of the liver is sought by exploring the postero-right edge of the portal vein in search of a right hepatic artery arising from the superior mesenteric artery, and by opening the lesser omentum in search of a left hepatic artery arising from the left gastric artery.
Depending on the proposed resection, an arterio-portal elective control can be prepared by placing the branches of the hepatic artery and portal vein on lakes.

### *(vii) Vascular clamping :*

The hepatic pedicle is clamped en masse, according to Pringle using a lac, placed around the hepatic pedicle, and subsequently inserted through a 16 F diameter rubber tube to act as a tourniquet during pedicle clamping. Clamping can be continuous or intermittent. Intermittent clamping is preferred in cases where clamping time is estimated to exceed 30 minutes, in cases of liver parenchymal abnormalities (steatosis, fibrosis, cirrhosis) and in cases of multiple resections. It consists of a 5-minute unclamp every 15 to 20 minutes. It is better tolerated than continuous clamping.
Whenever elective clamping can be envisaged (left lobectomy, right or left hepatectomy), it is performed and maintained in cases of satisfactory efficacy.
Complete vascular exclusion of the liver is used only in exceptional cases, and is reserved for voluminous centrohepatic metastases or metastases involving the dome of the liver or the inferior vena cava.

### *(viii) Parenchymal section:*

After incision of Glisson's capsule, parenchymal sectioning is performed using fine hemostatic forceps (Kellyclasie) or an ultrasonic scalpel. Accessory pedicles are either electrocoagulated with bipolar forceps, tied with 2/0 or 3/0 absorbable suture, or clipped progressively with locked absorbable clips. The main pedicles and suprahepatic veins are sutured, tied or, more rarely, stapled using an automatic vascular linear stapler.

### *(ix) Hepatectomy slice treatment:*

After unclamping, gentle compression of the hepatectomy slice is performed using abdominal drapes for a few minutes. Hemostasis is completed using thin crimped ligatures of 5/0 non-absorbable monofilament. Biliostasis is checked. Any biliary leaks are blinded with a fine suture of 5/0 absorbable monofilament.

### *(x) Drainage :*

Not systematically performed, using a multitubular blade or a drain placed at the level of Winslow's hiatus and externalized by a right counter-incision.

## 2. **Treatment by local destruction of liver metastases (TDLMH ):**

HSMT has developed recently, thanks in particular to advances in imaging, which is essential for its guidance. These techniques hold out great hope, including the possibility of destroying unresectable tumors, either in isolation or in association with surgery, or of reducing the burden of surgery by replacing all or part of it with HMLT. Today, the feasibility and tolerability of these techniques have only just been demonstrated, the local efficacy of each technique is still being evaluated, and only small series have been published. No study has rigorously compared these different techniques. What's more, rapid technological evolution, which is increasing the performance of the systems used, is rapidly rendering even recent results obsolete.

### *a) Radiofrequency ablation :*

### (1) Principle :

Radiofrequency ablation is the thermal destruction of tissue by circulating a high-frequency sinusoidal electric current (400 to 500 kHz) between one or more needle electrodes placed in the target tumor and dispersion plates placed on the patient's skin. This current induces ionic agitation in the tissues it passes through. Current density is high in regions close to the electrode, where this agitation causes significant tissue heating. The aim is to expose tumor cells to a temperature in excess of 60°C, leading almost immediately to irreversible cell denaturation.
On the other hand, it is not advisable to reach a temperature above the boiling point of the tissue, which, by releasing gas and carbonizing the tissue, increases its electrical resistance and alters the diffusion of the radiofrequency current, thus reducing the maximum size and homogeneity of the induced RF lesion.

### (2) Technology:

A bare, straight electrode induces a zone of tissue destruction with a diameter, perpendicular to the electrode, of no more than 1 to 1.5 cm. This is insufficient for the treatment of liver tumors. To increase the size of this destruction zone, several electrodes introduced through a single needle (deployable electrodes) are used, with needles containing several electrodes (4 to 12) which are then deployed in the target tumor. In this way, the number of destructions is equal to the number of electrodes, which are then spatially summed to form a single larger one. The size and shape of the final destruction zone depend, among other things, on the number of electrodes and their position in space.

### (a) Procedure:

Ultrasound provides real-time guidance.
Once the tumour has been located, the shortest route possible is chosen, avoiding extra-hepatic structures and the main hepatic vascular trunks if possible. The procedure is performed under strict conditions of surgical asepsis, including skin disinfection, sterile drapes and equipment (ultrasound probe in sterile cover, use of sterile gel).
Once the electrode(s) is/are in place, the radiofrequency current is delivered according to charts supplied by the manufacturer. Imaging detects numerous gas bubbles released by the heat.
At the end of the procedure, the electrodes are removed by coagulating the various puncture paths to limit the occurrence of hemorrhagic complications or tumor seeding of the puncture path. Post-treatment imaging is performed to ensure the absence of complications and to obtain an immediate post-therapeutic image of the target, which may prove useful for follow-up and evaluation of treatment efficacy.

### (b) Contraindications:

They share the same contraindications as hepatic puncture, with a few contraindications specific to the technique.

#### *(i) Contraindications to liver puncture :*

-Interposition of large vascular structures or the gall bladder on the puncture path.
-Dilatation of the bile ducts.
-Haemostasis disorders: a platelet count of at least 60000/mm$^3$ and a prothrombin level of over 50% are required for the procedure to be carried out. (112). Antiplatelet agents (clopidogrel, aspirin) and anticoagulants (antivitamin K, heparin) must be discontinued within a sufficiently short time.
-Medium to heavy ascites is a relative contraindication.

#### *(ii) Contraindications to radiofrequency treatment :*

-A bilio-digestive anastomosis is a relative contraindication due to the risk of post-radiofrequency sepsis.
-Proximity to the hilum, due to the risk of biliary stenosis.
-Proximity to the liver capsule is not a contraindication.
On the other hand, it makes the procedure more painful, and increases the intensity and duration of pain in the immediate aftermath of radiofrequency treatment.
-If the liver tumour comes into contact with, or is in close proximity to, the colon or stomach, there is a risk of digestive perforation. Such patients can be treated by injecting air or liquid to separate the target tumor from the hollow organs.

### (c) Indications :

Initially limited to the liver, radiofrequency indications in carcinology have naturally tended to extend to other organs.
For the treatment of primary or secondary liver tumors, radiofrequency can be used percutaneously or intraoperatively, during laparotomy or laparoscopy.
The high failure rate for tumors over 3 cm, due to the limitation of the size of the destruction zones to a maximum of 4 cm, means that this technique is reserved for small tumors. Tumors larger than 5 cm are virtually inaccessible to radiofrequency.

## 3. Laparoscopic approach:

The laparoscopic approach is a minimally invasive procedure, with advantages not only in terms of aesthetics, but also in terms of postoperative rehabilitation. Its contraindications are rare, but the risks associated with laparoscopy must be taken into account. These risks are mainly related to the creation of pneumoperitoneum, and the hemodynamic or respiratory consequences thereof.
Two types of complications can arise during the creation of pneumoperitoneum: digestive wounds and major vascular wounds. Digestive wounds are not immediately life-threatening. They occur in 0.5 to 0.8 ‰ of laparoscopies (113). In contrast, vascular wounds (particularly large-vessel wounds: aorta, vena cava, iliac vessels) are immediately life-threatening either because of the severity of the lesions, or because they are not immediately recognized. Their overall frequency is estimated at 0.4 ‰ (113).
Intraperitoneal insufflation of $CO_2$ has significant hemodynamic consequences, combining increased arterial pressure, reduced cardiac output and reduced venous return due to inferior vena cava compression. Under normal insufflation conditions, cardiac output is little affected. The situation is quite different in elderly patients and/or those with heart disease.
The perfusion of intra-abdominal organs during laparoscopy can be impaired by two phenomena, which are often associated: a drop in perfusion flow (which may depend on cardiac output as well as local conditions), and a drop in perfusion pressure.
Two types of respiratory effects can be identified during laparoscopic surgery: those related to the systemic passage of insufflated $CO_2$ and those related to intraperitoneal insufflation.
The hypercapnia induced at the start of the procedure (and which may persist after exsufflation) can induce deleterious metabolic acidosis (arterial hypertension, intracranial hypertension, cardiac rhythm disorders) and must be compensated by alveolar hyperventilation.

Laparoscopic surgery, a fortiori in the declive position, induces a drop in diaphragmatic compliance, resulting in a 30-50% reduction in total pulmonary compliance.

Also, intraperitoneal insufflation of dry, unheated gas, as well as washing with cold fluids, leads to caloric loss during laparoscopic surgery (intraoperative hypothermia).
Other complications include capnic gas embolism, a classic complication of laparoscopic surgery, favored by accidental intravascular insufflation or the opening of veins in the surgical site. Other complications include intracranial and intraocular hypertension.

### *a) Colorectal cancer:*

Laparoscopic colorectal resection has been shown to be safe and effective in several large randomized trials, and has gained acceptance as an alternative to the conventional route. The minimally invasive nature of laparoscopic surgery improves comfort and reduces the rate of postoperative complications. Laparoscopy reduces postoperative pain (less parietal trauma), and has a positive effect on postoperative ileus and respiratory function. It also reduces intraoperative stress and, consequently, postoperative immunodepression. Hospital stay is shorter, and the return to normal activity is quicker, with an overall better quality of life for the patient. Alongside these advantages, laparoscopy is carcinologically effective and safe in selected patients, despite the additional cost of the surgical procedure.

### *b) Liver metastases :*

Since the first laparoscopic liver resection in 1992 by M.Gagner (24)laparoscopic liver surgery has continued to develop, offering the same advantages as colorectal surgery, with less morbidity, less pain, faster recovery, shorter hospital stay than open procedures, without compromising oncological clearance. Several expert consensus conferences have been organized, in Louisville in 2008 and Morioka in 2014 (114) which concluded that minor liver resections were standard practice under laparoscopy, notably left lobectomy (Gold standard).

Major resections remained under development in expert centers. In 2017, the first European recommendations concerning laparoscopic liver surgery were published (115) which pointed in the same direction, paving the way for a better codified practice of laparoscopic liver surgery.

The results of the first randomized controlled trial comparing laparoscopic surgery for liver metastases and conventional surgery were published in 2018, the rate of postoperative complications was lower in the laparoscopic arm (116).

In 2018 M.C.Halls et al (117) published a difficulty score to predict intraoperative complications specific to laparoscopic liver surgery.
This score assigns points to five risk factors used in the predictive model to estimate the risk of intraoperative complications during laparoscopic liver resections (table 5, table 6).

**Table 5** Risk of complications (Halls score) (117).

| Risk factor | Risk factor category | Points assigned |
|---|---|---|
| Neoadjuvant chemotherapy | No | 0 |
| | Yes | 1 |
| Previous open liver resection | No | 0 |
| | Yes | 5 |
| Lesion type | Benign | 0 |
| | Malignant | 2 |
| Lesion size (cm) | < 3 | 0 |
| | 3–5 | 2 |
| | > 5 | 3 |
| Classification of resection | Minor | 0 |
| | Technically major | 2 |
| | Anatomically major | 4 |

Points for each of the five risk factors were assigned as described in Table 5, and summed to give a total score. Low-risk procedures are suitable for surgeons at the beginning of the learning curve. Moderate-risk procedures are suitable only for surgeons who have overcome the learning curve for minor resections. High-risk procedures are suitable only for surgeons who have overcome the learning curve for minor and major resections. Procedures considered extremely high-risk should only be performed by leaders in the field.

**Table 6** Risk assessment using the Halls score (117).

| Total points scored | Post-calibration risk | Risk group |
|---|---|---|
| 0 | 0·5 | Low |
| 1 | 3·0 | Low |
| 2 | 6·1 | Low |
| 3 | 9·9 | Moderate |
| 4 | 14·5 | Moderate |
| 5 | 20·0 | Moderate |
| 6 | 26·2 | High |
| 7 | 33·1 | High |
| 8 | 40·3 | High |
| 9 | 47·6 | High |
| 10 | 54·7 | Extremely high |
| 11 | 61·3 | Extremely high |
| 12 | 69·8 | Extremely high |
| 13 | 72·4 | Extremely high |
| 14 | 76·7 | Extremely high |
| 15 | 80·2 | Extremely high |

In 2019 Ruben Ciria (118)reported different difficulty scores for laparoscopic liver surgery. The difficulty factors individualized by 11 authors are summarized in Table 7.

These factors are related to the patient, liver function and type of surgery.

**Table 7** Difficulty scores for laparoscopic liver surgery (118).

| Difficulty scores in laparoscopic liver surgery | | Troisi | Ban | Cauchy | Lee | Wakabayashi | Hasegawa | Halls | Silva | Kawaguchy | Tong | Tong |
|---|---|---|---|---|---|---|---|---|---|---|---|---|
| | | 2014 | 2014 | 2015 | 2015 | 2016 | 2017 | 2018 | 2018 | 2018 | 2019 | 2019 |
| Patient status | Age | | | | | | | | | | | |
| | Diabetes | | | | | | | | | | | |
| | BMI | | | | | | | | | | | |
| | Hypertension | | | | | | | | | | | |
| | Previous open liver resection | | | | | | | | | | | |
| | Neoadjuvant chemotherapy | | | | | | | | | | | |
| | ASA score | | | | | | | | | | | |
| Liver status | Liver function | | | | | | | | | | | |
| | Platelet count | | | | | | | | | | | |
| | ALT | | | | | | | | | | | |
| Technical terms | Extent of liver resection | | | | | | | | | | | |
| | Tumor location | | | | | | | | | | | |
| | Proximity to major vessels | | | | | | | | | | | |
| | Biliary reconstruction | | | | | | | | | | | |
| | Tumor size | | | | | | | | | | | |
| | HALS/hybrid | | | | | | | | | | | |
| | Operative time | | | | | | | | | | | |
| | Pathology | | | | | | | | | | | |
| Maximum scoring | | – | 10 | – | 10 | 12 | 7 | 15 | – | 3 | 6 | 13 |
| Subclassification | | – | Low: 0–3<br>Intermediate: 4–6<br>High: 7–10 | – | Low<br>Medium<br>High | Low: 0–3<br>Intermediate: 4–6<br>Advanced: 7–9<br>Expert: 10–12 | Low: 0–1<br>Medium: 2–3<br>High: 4–more | Low: 0–2<br>Moderate: 3–5<br>High: 6–9<br>Extremely high: 10–15 | – | I: 0 points<br>II: 2 points<br>III: 3 points | Low ≤1<br>Medium =2<br>High ≥3 | Low 0–1<br>Medium 2–4<br>High ≥5 |
| Comments | | No risk categories | Iwate score, further validated | No risk categories | Extension-only score | Update of Ban 2014 | | Southampton score | No risk categories | A posteriori score | | |
| Endpoint variable | | Conversion | Degree of difficulty | Conversion | Degree of difficulty | Degree of difficulty | Degree of difficulty | Intraoperative complications | Conversion | Degree of difficulty | Conversion | Complication |

# VI. Materials and methods:

## A. Study design :

### 1. Objectives :

The aim of the study was to assess the **feasibility and safety** of the laparoscopic approach in **combined surgery** for colorectal cancer with synchronous liver metastases.

Scientific hypothesis:

Our study hypothesis was as follows:
**The laparoscopic approach to the combined management of colorectal cancer with synchronous liver metastases** is feasible, with a morbi-mortality rate that **is no higher than** that **of the laparoscopic** approach **to colorectal cancer alone**, and a low conversion rate. It is safe **from a carcinological** standpoint (quality of excision, recurrence rate and survival), and at the same time offers an advantage in terms of the quality of post-operative **rehabilitation.**

The objectives of the study were:

Principal :

- Evaluate postoperative morbidity and mortality at 30 days.
  - Judging criteria :
    - Morbidity <30
    - Mortality < 5%.
    - No significant increase in morbidity and mortality compared with the control arm.

Secondary :

- Calculate conversion rate (TConv): judgement criterion TConv < 15%.
- Evaluate the quality of exeresis.
- Evaluate post-operative rehabilitation and quality of life (pain, post-operative stay, resumption of eating, resumption of transit).
- Calculate the recurrence rate.
- Calculate 3-year survival rate (overall and recurrence-free).

## 2. Study protocol :

### a) *Type of study :*

Longitudinal, prospective, comparative intervention study.

### b) *Study population :*

**Experimental arm :**

Patients presenting with CCRMHS for whom the initial therapeutic objective was curative, undergoing simultaneous laparoscopic surgery on at least one of the two tumor sites (colorectal/hepatic).

**Control arm :**

Contemporary cohort of patients undergoing laparoscopic colorectal cancer surgery during the same study period.

### c) *Sample size :*

To meet the objectives of our study, we had to select patients with a double filter: the curative objective and management at the beginning of the therapeutic pathway, thus excluding second-hand patients (e.g. primary tumor already operated on and patient admitted for treatment of synchronous liver metastases) and patients with a palliative strategy. The rarity of the clinical presentation taken as the object of our study, verified by the data in the literature as presented previously, obliged us to define a study sample compatible with our local statistics.

In our department, we manage around 15 patients a year who could be included in our study.

On the duration of the study, which included a phase of patient inclusion, therapeutic management, data collection and analysis, and finally writing up the results. We conducted a study on a sample of **N = 40** patients.

### d) *Study duration: 41 months*

Data was collected on an individual data sheet for each patient (Appendix 1), then entered into an Excel file.

## e) *Inclusion :*

**Experimental arm :**

Inclusion criteria:

1. Age > 18 and < 80.
2. Resectable adenocarcinoma of the rectum or colon.
3. Synchronous hepatic metastasis(es) confirmed on MRI and/or CT deemed resectable after RCP evaluation.
4. Absence of other unresectable metastatic sites.
5. Normal haematological, hepatic and renal tests.
6. Karnofsky Index ≥ 70, WHO Performance Index ≤ 2.
7. Informed consent.

Non-inclusion criteria:

1. Age ≤18 years and ≥ 80years.
2. Pregnant or breast-feeding women.
3. History of malignant tumor within 5 years.
4. Karnofsky Index < 70, WHO Performance Index > 2.
5. Contraindication to surgery.
6. Discovery of unresectable metastases in other organs.
7. Mental disorders.

**Control arm :**

Inclusion criteria:

1. Age > 18 years and < 80 years.
2. resectable adenocarcinoma of the rectum or colon.
3 Normal haematological, hepatic and renal tests.
4. Karnofsky index ≥ 70, WHO performance index ≤ 2.
5. informed consent.
6. Operated by the same surgeon (on the experimental arm).

Non-inclusion criteria:

1. Age ≤18 years and ≥ 80years.
2 Pregnant or breast-feeding women.
3. history of malignant tumour within 5 years.

4 Karnofsky index < 70, WHO performance index > 2.
5 Contraindication to surgery.
6 Mental disorders.

**Defining the therapeutic strategy :**

For each case included, the therapeutic strategy was decided at the start of management, after discussion at a multidisciplinary consultation meeting (RCP). The order and interval between the different therapeutic modalities (chemotherapy, radiotherapy and surgery) were specified.

The laparoscopic approach to combined surgery could take several forms:
1-The laparoscopic approach: the primary tumor and liver metastasis were removed laparoscopically.

2-Hybrid surgery: a combination of laparoscopic and conventional approaches to two distinct tumor sites.

3-Laparoscopic ˝down staging˝ surgery: part of the two-stage hepatectomy for patients with multiple bilobar metastases, either :

3.1 Laparoscopic resection of the primary tumor + laparoscopic portal ligation +/- laparoscopic surgery of liver metastases on one hemi-lumen followed by a second major hepatectomy via the conventional route.

3.2 First hybrid resection (laparoscopic resection of the primary tumor combined with resection of part of the hepatic metastases), followed by surgery to remove the rest of the hepatic metastases by conventional means.

### *f) Comparison :*

Patients in the two study arms were matched on the basis of the following preoperative variables: age, gender, ASA grade, neoadjuvant radiotherapy, primary tumor location, type of colorectal resection and T and N stage of the primary tumor . Results were compared using paired tests.

## 3. Pre-therapy evaluation :

Patient files were discussed at a multidisciplinary consultation meeting (RCP) to define the treatment modalities and the chronology of action of the various parties involved (oncologist, surgeon, radiotherapist, etc.), but beforehand an exhaustive clinical and paraclinical assessment was carried out.

### *a) Clinical evaluation :*

Performed in consultation. Personal and family history was taken (comorbidities, risk factors, neoplastic history, history of abdominal surgery, etc.).
It specified the reason for consultation, the date of symptom onset and the evolution of symptoms.
A complete physical examination assessed general condition (WHO performance index), nutritional status and calculated BMI.
Examination of the digestive system was to include a rectal examination.
The lymph nodes were systematically examined.
Abdominal scarring was noted.
Classification of patients according to the American Society of Anesthesiologists (ASA) classification for anesthetic risk assessment.

### *b) Paraclinical evaluation :*

Had a dual objective: to assess the patient and the disease.

**Diagnosis and extension :**
Lower digestive endoscopy with biopsy to establish the diagnosis.
In the case of rectal tumors, pelvic MRI was performed.
In the case of colonic or rectal tumors, a three-phase thoraco-abdomino-pelvic CT scan was performed to assess extension, and to determine the topography, number, volume and vascular relationships of hepatic metastases and the state of the liver parenchyma. Liver volumetry was performed if required.
Hepatic MRI was performed in addition to CT for better lesion characterization.
A total colonoscopy was performed when the tumor could be crossed, in search of synchronous localizations (polyp, tumor).
In the event of an impassable tumour, a colonoscan was performed.
Tumor markers were assayed, in particular ACE and CA19.9.
Determination of tumor RAS gene status (*KRAS and NRAS*) on primary tumor or metastatic tissue.

**Operability:**
In addition to the clinical assessment of vital functions and comorbidities, the pre-anaesthesia consultation evaluated the data from the biological workup:

- Blood count
- Blood grouping
- Uremia, creatininemia, glycemia.
- Prothrombin level.
- Transaminases, alkaline phosphatases, gamma glutamyl transferase, bilirubins.
- Albumin levels, protein levels
- Blood ionogram.

And cardiac electrical (ECG) and ultrasonographic tests.

## 4. **Treatment strategy :**

Patients included in the study were candidates for simultaneous surgery, with laparoscopic approach to at least one tumor site scheduled.

Different treatment modalities were proposed by the RCP, depending on the location of the primary tumor (colon, rectum), whether liver metastases were resectable (class I) or potentially resectable (class II), their number, location (anterior or posterior segments) and whether they were bilobar or unilobar.

Rectal primitive :

Depending on tumor location (upper/middle and lower rectum) and stage, the indication for neoadjuvant treatment was discussed.

For cancers of the middle or lower rectum T1-T2 N0 or for tumors of the upper rectum, by analogy with a non-metastatic situation, there is no indication for preoperative treatment.

For locally advanced tumors of the middle or lower rectum (T3 and/or N+) not resectable R0 from the outset, i.e. with a predictable circumferential margin on MRI of less than 1 mm. Preoperative RCT was indicated.

In the case of T3 or N+ cancers with R0 resectability, i.e. CRM > 1 mm on MRI, short radiotherapy was feasible.

Where indicated, chemotherapy for liver metastases was performed before RT in the case of a short protocol.

In summary, the type of neoadjuvant treatment depended on predictable resection margins and the extent of metastatic disease.

Several options were available:

- Short course radiotherapy/immediate combined surgery.
- Short course radiotherapy/deferred combined surgery.
- Concomitant radiochemotherapy/combined surgery deferred.

Primitive colonic :

Or combined surgery from the outset, in the case of a single small liver metastasis.

Or combined surgery preceded by intraoperative or neoadjuvant chemotherapy, depending on whether the liver metastases are resectable or potentially resectable.

Special case of two-stage hepatectomy:

Chemotherapy + targeted therapy followed by resection of the primary tumor combined with a liver procedure consisting of either :

- Portal ligation +/- clearance of a half-liver.
- Partial resection of liver metastases.

A second hepatic step was scheduled after an interval, and volumetry was reassessed if a portal ligation had been performed during the first step.

In the meantime, chemotherapy was reintroduced.

## 5. Processing :

### *a) Drug treatment :*

When chemotherapy was indicated, the protocol depended on the resectability class of liver metastases (Appendix 2).

**In case of class I resectability :**
- FOLFOX 4 simplifies: 4 to 6 preoperative courses and 6 to 8 postoperative courses.
- CAPOX: 3 preoperative courses and 5 postoperative courses.

Total of six months of pre- and post-operative treatment.

**In case of class II resectability :**
Biochemotherapy plus biotherapy:
Biochemotherapy combined with Cetuximab or Panitumumab in the absence of RAS mutation, or bichimiotherapy combined with Bevacizumab.

### *b) Radiotherapy:*

#### (1) Concomitant radiochemotherapy:

-Protocol ≪ CAP 50 ≫ :
- 50 Gy in 25 fractions spread over 5 weeks (2 Gy per fraction),
- Concomitant chemotherapy: Capecitabine (1,600 mg/m2 divided into 1 morning and evening dose of 800 mg/m2 on radiotherapy days).
- Time to surgical resection: 7 ± 1 weeks after completion of RT.

-Long radiotherapy: 45 - 50 Gy /25 - 28 Fractions/5 weeks combined with FUFOL (standard): 5-Fluorouracil (350mg/m2/day) + Folinic acid (20mg/day), delivered during the first five (05) days of the first and fifth week of irradiation.

#### (2) Short course radiotherapy :

- 25Gy /5Fractions/ 5 days.

### *c) Surgery:*

**Preparing the patient for surgery :**
Patients were systematically included in the AGER (Algerian Group of Enhanced recovery) enhanced rehabilitation protocol introduced in the department since 2017 for patients with colorectal cancer (appendix 3).
Patient information was an important part of the protocol (information on the pathology, the operating procedure, the possibility of a stoma, pain management, post-operative rehabilitation, etc.).
Colonic preparation (oral preparation, enema and/or residue-free diet) was reserved for patients with rectal tumors.

For those with colonic tumors, mechanical preparation by Wash-out was not performed, but the residue-free diet was prescribed.
Patients received thromboprophylaxis and antibiotic prophylaxis.
Patients were given a sugary drink 2 to 3 hours before the procedure.
Perioperative management :

**Immediate preoperative care:**
Welcoming the patient to the operating room was an important stage (psychological preparation with preoperative information helps to reduce postoperative analgesic consumption and shorten hospital stay).
Systematic prescription of anxiolytic premedication was outlawed, and psychological support with explanations and de-dramatization from the consultation onwards was vital.
In our department, premedication was non-pharmacological.
Prevention of postoperative nausea and vomiting was systematically combined according to the Apfel score (appendix 4): Dexamethasone 8mg for prevention, and ondansetron 4mg for cure.
Muscle relaxants were administered as required and monitored by a curarometer.
Antibiotic prophylaxis was adapted according to the AGER protocol (appendix 3).
Since hemodynamic stability is essential for a smooth postoperative course, a syringe of ephedrine was prepared to avoid any drop in blood pressure due to vasodilatation from hypnotics and associated analgesia, such as epidurals or TAP Bloc ( transverse abdominal plane block ) under ultrasound guidance.
The patient's welcome began with an introduction to the team, as serene communication from the outset is often a prerequisite for positive patient behavior.
The patient's identity and ASA score were verified on the anesthesia sheet in a non-stressful way.
In the absence of diabetes and delayed gastric emptying, the patient had already drunk a sugar-rich herbal tea 2 to 3 h before arriving at the operating theatre.
The patient was actively positioned on the operating table and warmed up with a warm air blanket (warming up is one of the protocol's priorities).
Hypothermia is responsible for a reduced immune response, delayed healing and abscess formation, increased coagulation disorders and increased cardiovascular morbidity in the recovery and postoperative phases. The HAS (Haute autorité de santé) checklist was checked in the presence of all those involved.

**Period of operation :**
The use of short-acting general anesthetic agents shortens the recovery period.
Locoregional analgesia (LRA) was favored from the intraoperative period: epidural analgesia, peripheral TAP Blocs or infiltration of wound edges with local anesthetics.
Pulsed hot-air blankets were re-installed in an optimal way, seeking the best compromise between the best possible heating and surgical imperatives.
Thrombosis was systematically prevented with isocoagulant LMWH.

In the case of obesity, the dose of antibiotic prophylaxis was doubled and the prescription of isocoagulant-dose LMWH was increased to twice daily, in accordance with the recommendations of the French Society of Intensive Care Anaesthesia (119,120).
More or less invasive hemodynamic monitoring depending on the patient, with central catheter placement and/or blood pressure (BP) to optimize vascular filling, was performed according to comorbidities.
Temperature was monitored. The thermal probe was inserted through the mouth to avoid any untimely nasal lesions, and eye protection was carefully applied.
Vascular approaches were preferentially peripheral, with central catheterization indicated according to the patient's ASA classification to guide vascular filling.

Preoxygenation was carried out in a participatory and active manner, with the patient providing inspiratory support to achieve 90% FiO2 for better apnea tolerance.
Trendelenburg positioning was systematic in obese or overweight patients (deckchair position).
The ventilator was set according to the ideal weight for tidal volume (6 to 8 ml/kg), respiratory rate was set according to exhaled CO2 and positive expiratory pressure (PEEP) between 8 and 10 cmH2O was systematically applied.
The recommended FiO2 was around 60% for good tissue oxygenation. Regular alveolar recruitment maneuvers to avoid atelectasis were repeated.
Throughout the operative period, curarization was monitored to facilitate the surgical procedure.

Basic hydration was 4ml/kg/h, and vascular filling was adapted according to central venous pressure (CVP), in order to avoid deleterious inadequate volumes, which considerably increase postoperative complications such as renal failure in the case of hypovolaemia, and overload with oedema and risk of fistula and prolonged ileus in the case of hypervolaemia. A gastric tube was inserted, but systematically removed at the end of the procedure.
Glycemic monitoring was carried out in diabetics, and gasometry was performed in all patients.

Postoperative analgesia began 30 min before closure, and was multimodal, giving preference to intravenous non-morphine agents (paracetamol, nefopam).
If an epidural was in place, a reinjection bolus was also performed at this time.

Ventilatory weaning was usually performed in the operating room with spontaneous ventilation with inspiratory support, and curare antagonization was performed after checking the "Train of 4" (TOF).
Decurarization is only confirmed after 4 responses with a T1/T4 ratio > 95%.
A mouth suction was performed in the still-asleep patient, and an alveolar recruitment maneuver performed immediately afterwards to re-expand the lungs.

**Post-operative period:** in the post-operative monitoring room (SSPI).

Pain was monitored using the VAS at rest and on exertion, and if an epidural was in place, the epidural level was assessed using the cold test.
Despite prevention with dexamethasone during induction, if postoperative nausea and vomiting occurred, ondansetron 4 mg was the curative treatment used in our protocol.
The patient was evacuated to the ward according to the modified ALDRETE score (appendix 5).

The operating procedure was divided into three stages:

The first stage was laparoscopic abdominal exploration to rule out peritoneal carcinosis. The second step was laparoscopic colorectal resection, followed by a third step, resection of the liver metastasis, performed either laparoscopically or by open surgery via a right subcostal incision with or without a median subxiphoid slit, or via a short midline incision.

In the case of laparoscopic resection of the liver metastasis, extraction of both parts (colorectal and liver) was performed via a Pfannenstiel incision.

In the case of open liver resection, the colorectal resection specimen was extracted through the abdominal incision chosen for liver resection, depending on the site of liver metastases and the patient's anatomy.

**At the end of the intervention :**

Intraoperative incidents were recorded.
The operating time was recorded.

## (1) Surgery of the primary tumor: (see video 1)

Installation of the patient and surgical team :
The procedure was performed under general anaesthesia. In the case of a rectal primary, digital rectal examination (DRE) under general anaesthetic was performed systematically.
The patient was positioned in the double-team position, with arms alongside the body, and urinary catheterization was performed sterilely before the surgical drapes were applied. The position of the surgical team depended on the tumour location: in the case of a left colonic or rectal tumour, the operator was positioned on the patient's right, the first assistant responsible for the camera on the surgeon's left, the second assistant between the patient's legs; in the case of a right colonic tumour, the operator was positioned on the patient's left, the first assistant on the surgeon's right, the second assistant between the patient's legs.
The pneumoperitoneum was created using a Veress needle or open laparoscopy. The pressure of the pneumoperitoneum was preset at 12 mm of mercury. Trocars were positioned according to the site of the primary tumor.

In the case of a left colonic tumour, four trocars were used: an 11 mm umbilical optical trocar, and three operating trocars (12 mm trocar in the right iliac fossa, 05 mm trocar on the left flank, 05 mm trocar on the right hypochondrium).
In the case of rectal tumours, a fifth trocar was inserted suprapubically.
In the case of a right colonic tumour, four trocars were used: an 11 mm umbilical optical trocar, and three operating trocars (12 mm trocar in the left hypochondrium, 05 mm trocar in the left iliac fossa, 05 mm trocar in the right iliac fossa).

The procedure began with laparoscopic exploration of the various diaphragms, in search of possible peritoneal carcinosis. This time was used to determine the characteristics of the primary tumor and hepatic metastases (use of a 30° optic for hepatic exploration).
If there were no contraindications to resection, the procedure was continued.
The patient was tilted into the Trendelenburg position with a lateral roll opposite the tumor topography.

Laparoscopic colorectal resection was performed in compliance with carcinological rules.
In the case of a left colonic or rectal primary:
First proximal ligation of inferior mesenteric vessels, inferior mesenteric artery 1 cm from its origin respecting the superior hypogastric plexus, and inferior mesenteric vein at the inferior edge of the pancreas, coloparietal detachment via the medial approach, complete mobilization of the splenic angle. In the case of a left colonic tumour, distal section was performed with a 60 mm mechanical stapler at promontory level.
In the case of rectal tumors, partial or total resection of the mesorectum was combined. Rectal dissection reaches 5 cm below the lower edge of the tumour for tumours of the upper rectum, and reaches the pelvic floor for tumours of the middle and lower rectum.
Distal sectioning was performed with a 45mm mechanical cutting stapler.
Continuity was re-established by mechanical anastomosis (colorectal or colo-sus-anal anastomosis) using circular forceps, or manual colo-anal anastomosis, depending on tumour location. The anastomosis was protected by a lateral ileostomy positioned at the level of the trocar orifice in the right iliac fossa in the case of subperitoneal anastomosis.
A left iliac colostomy was performed in case of abdominoperineal amputation.
For cancers of the right colon, vessel ligation was performed to the right of the superior mesenteric axis, followed by complete mobilization of the right colon from medial to lateral, with anastomosis performed extracorporeally through a right transverse incision subsequently used for the hepatic phase.
Drainage was not systematic.

### (2) Liver metastasis surgery:

In combined surgery, the hepatic approach had several objectives: firstly, exhaustive exploration of hepatic metastases (visual, ultrasound, palpatory if approached by laparotomy); then, if the indication was maintained after this exploration stage, a carcinological excision or thermoablation procedure was carried out; it was possible to associate a portal ligation within the framework of two-stage hepatectomies.

This hepatic surgery could be performed either via a laparoscopic approach or a conventional approach in association with the laparoscopic procedure on the primary tumor.

The chronological order in the operative procedure between the liver and colorectal resection was decided on a case-by-case basis.

### (a) Laparoscopic liver surgery :

The laparoscopic approach to liver metastases required an additional trocar in the epigastric position (Fig.26). Others could be placed on request.

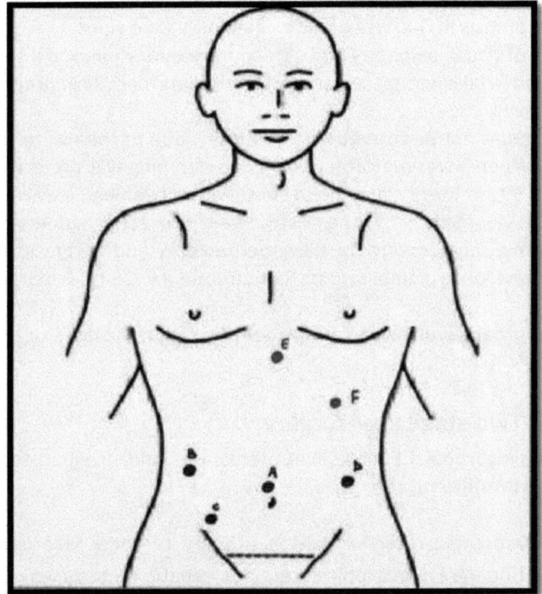


**Figure 26** Trocar layout for combined laparoscopic surgery (121).
(Blue A,B,C,D trocars for colorectal time, red E and/or F additional trocars for liver time).

Hepatic clamping was prepared by placing a lake around the hepatic pedicle, which was put on hold.

Laparoscopic liver resection could be metastasectomy, atypical resection or minor (<3 segments) regulated resection with or without clamping.

After laparoscopic exploration and identification of lesions, definition of resection margins and, if necessary, pedicle control, parenchymal transsection was

performed using a combination of different energy sources: ultrasound (CUSA and ultracision), electricity (bipolar), clips and mechanical sutures for glissonian and vascular pedicles.
If indicated, laparoscopic portal ligation was performed using locked clips.
Extraction was performed in a bag through a Pfannenstiel incision.
Drainage was not systematic.
The laparoscopic approach was preferred for small, superficial liver metastases located in accessible anteroinferior segments (II, III, IVb, V and VI).

### (b) Combined liver surgery by laparotomy: (hybrid approach)

Laparotomy for liver metastases was also used to extract the colorectal resection specimen and prepare the colonic transplant for anastomosis (e.g., anvil placement), in the case of anterior or left colonic resection, or as a route for ileocolic anastomosis in the case of right colectomy (See video 1).
After a period of visual, palpatory and ultrasound exploration, and if the indication was maintained, a lake was placed around the hepatic pedicle in preparation for a Pringle maneuver.
Liver clamping was not performed systematically, due to the risk to the digestive anastomosis. When it was performed, selective clamping was preferred to pedicle clamping, and intermittent clamping to continuous clamping.
Less than 3 segments of the liver were resected (minor resection). Metastasectomy, segmentectomy, bisegmentectomy and wedge resection were performed alone or in combination. Radiofrequency thermoablation could be performed.
The hybrid approach was preferred for deep, large metastases in the posterior segments (VII, VIII, IVa and I).

### (c) Two-stage liver surgery:

Indicated for synchronous bilobar liver metastases and/or when the remaining liver volume is insufficient.
It could be :

- Laparoscopic resection of the primary tumor + laparoscopic portal ligation +/- laparoscopic surgery of hepatic metastases on one hemi-lumen followed by a second major hepatectomy via the conventional route.
- A first hybrid resection (laparoscopic resection of the primary tumor combined with resection of part of the hepatic metastases) followed by surgery to remove the rest of the hepatic metastases by conventional means.

## 6. Conversion :

We considered **conversion** to be the necessity of performing the entire surgical procedure (colorectal and liver times) by laparotomy.

## 7. **Pathological anatomy :**

After surgical resection, the surgical specimens were measured, the margins checked and the integrity of the mesorectum assessed in the case of proctectomy. Specimens were then sent fresh to the pathological anatomy department of the Pierre & Marie Curie Center for analysis, accompanied by an explanatory sheet.
The results of the analysis were later received in the form of a report which included the macroscopic, histological, immunohistochemical and molecular study of the surgical specimen.

### *a) Macroscopic examination :*

All the following elements were specified:
Packaging the surgical part.

For the colorectal resection specimen:
The dimensions of the specimen, the size of the tumor, the distance between the tumor and the nearest resection limit, the appearance of the tumor, the percentage of circumferential invasion, the confirmation or otherwise of perforation in the tumor zone, the presence of nodules of carcinosis and other possible lesions, and the appearance of the mesorectum according to the classification of Quirke et al. (64).

For the hepatectomy specimen:
The dimensions of the part, the appearance of the nodule when cut and the nearest resection limit.

### *b) Microscopic examination :*

All the following elements were specified:

Histological type.
The grade according to the WHO 2010 classification (table 2).
Depth extension (or infiltration level) classified according to the latest version of the pTNM classification (8$^{ème}$ edition).
In the case of neoadjuvant treatment, whether radiotherapy, chemotherapy, targeted therapy or their combination, the prefix "y" was added.

Histological response to neoadjuvant treatment :
Response to neoadjuvant therapy was assessed using the RCRG classification for the primary tumor and the TRG (Rubbia Brandt) classification for the secondary tumor. (66) for liver metastases (table 8).
Surgical resection limits :
The integrity or invasiveness of the proximal and distal surgical resection limits were mentioned.
For rectal tumors in non-peritoneal areas, the circumferential margin or clearance was specified.

Extension :
- Nodes: The number of nodes removed and the number of metastatic nodes were specified.
- Adventitial nodules : The existence of adventitial nodules or satellite nodules located in the pericolic or perirectal tissue was noted.
- Vasculolymphatic emboli :
- Perineural infiltration :

Tumor extension was classified according to the pTNM classification (8$^{ème}$ edition, 2017 of AJCC) and stage was specified according to UICC stages.

Liver toxicity :
Post-chemotherapy hepatic lesions were investigated, namely the existence of possible irinotecan-related steatohepatitis or oxaliplatin-related vascular lesions of sinusoid obstruction syndrome (or SOS syndrome).

Molecular factors :
MSI, BRAF and RAS statuses were specified.

**Table 8** Tumor regression grade classifications used, RCRG classification for primary tumor, TRG classification for liver metastases (122).

| | |
|---|---|
| Original RCRG system | |
| RCRG 1 | Sterilization or only microscopic foci of adenocarcinoma remaining, with marked fibrosis |
| RCRG 2 | Marked fibrosis but macroscopic disease present |
| RCRG 3 | Little or no fibrosis, with abundant macroscopic disease |
| m-RCRG system | |
| m-RCRG 1 | The macroscopic features may be varied. Microscopy reveals no tumour epithelium or scattered foci of malignant epithelium comprising < 5% of the overall area of abnormality. Mucin pools may be present but do not contain malignant epithelium |
| m-RCRG 2 | The macroscopic features may be varied. Microscopy reveals a combination of viable tumour epithelium and fibrosis. Malignant epithelium comprises 5–50% of the overall area of abnormality |
| m-RCRG 3 | The macroscopic and microscopic features may not be significantly different to cases in which neoadjuvant therapy has not been given. Over 50% of the area of abnormality comprises malignant epithelium. Some fibrosis may be present but no more than that commonly seen as desmoplastic stroma in cases where no neoadjuvant therapy has been given |
| TRG system | |
| TRG 1 | No viable cancer cells |
| TRG 2 | Single cells or small groups of cancer cells |
| TRG 3 | Residual cancer outgrown by fibrosis |
| TRG 4 | Significant fibrosis outgrown by cancer |
| TRG 5 | No fibrosis with extensive residual cancer |

## 8. Perioperative adverse events:

### *a) Intraoperative :*

Evaluated by the Oslo classification (123) which modified Satava's (124) dealing with intraoperative incidents (Fig.27).

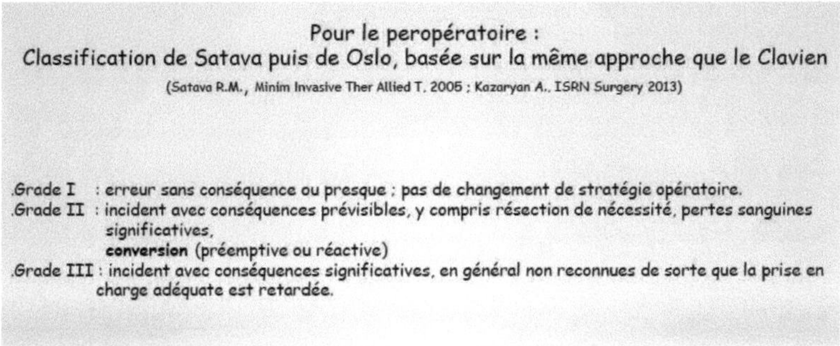

Pour le peropératoire :
Classification de Satava puis de Oslo, basée sur la même approche que le Clavien
(Satava R.M., Minim Invasive Ther Allied T. 2005 ; Kazaryan A., ISRN Surgery 2013)

.Grade I : erreur sans conséquence ou presque ; pas de changement de stratégie opératoire.
.Grade II : incident avec conséquences prévisibles, y compris résection de nécessité, pertes sanguines significatives,
**conversion** (préemptive ou réactive)
.Grade III : incident avec conséquences significatives, en général non reconnues de sorte que la prise en charge adéquate est retardée.

**Figure 27** Oslo classification (123).

### *b) Immediate postoperative follow-up :*

Post-operatively, the patient could be transferred to an intensive care unit or an inpatient unit (the intensive care stay was recorded).
The multimodal analgesia protocol was recorded on the anesthesia record on leaving the operating room.
A daily clinical examination was carried out, and a systematic biological check-up was requested on D01 and D03 postoperatively (CBC, blood count, uremia, creatininemia, liver function tests, ionogram, albumin level). A check-up at D00 could be performed on a case-by-case basis.
The urinary catheter was removed at D01, and the surgeon decided to remove the drainage.
The patient woke up early, between D00 and D01 postoperatively.
Liquid feeding was allowed from day 00 in the absence of nausea or vomiting.
The date on which transit was resumed was recorded, and postoperative pain was assessed on D01 postoperatively using a visual analog scale (VAS).
Discharge was decided on the basis of a normal clinical examination of an apyretic, autonomous patient who was able to eat and had resumed transit. In the absence of pain, nausea or vomiting, with a correct biological check-up.
The length of the postoperative stay was recorded on the patient's chart.

### *c) Mortality :*

was assessed at 30 days, and the cause of death in this eventuality was specified.

### d) *Morbidity :*

Evaluated at 30 days, events could occur during hospitalization or after discharge. Any readmission to our department or to another health facility was noted. Severity of morbidity was assessed according to the Clavien-Dindo-Strasberg classification (125,126) (Fig. 28).

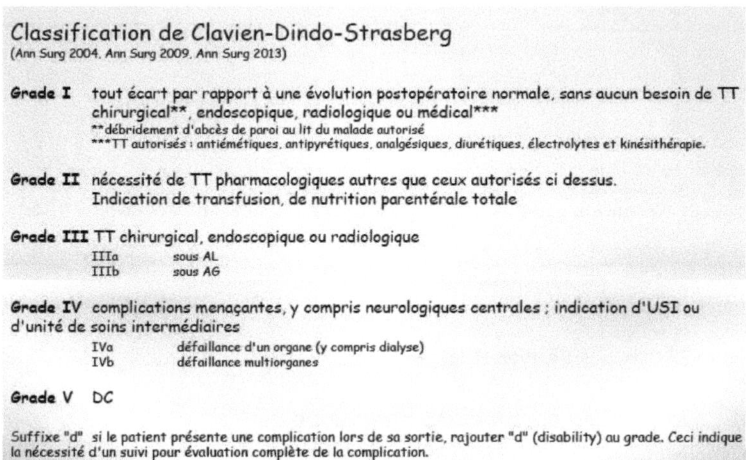

Classification de Clavien-Dindo-Strasberg
(Ann Surg 2004, Ann Surg 2009, Ann Surg 2013)

**Grade I** tout écart par rapport à une évolution postopératoire normale, sans aucun besoin de TT chirurgical**, endoscopique, radiologique ou médical***
**débridement d'abcès de paroi au lit du malade autorisé
***TT autorisés : antiémétiques, antipyrétiques, analgésiques, diurétiques, électrolytes et kinésithérapie.

**Grade II** nécessité de TT pharmacologiques autres que ceux autorisés ci dessus.
Indication de transfusion, de nutrition parentérale totale

**Grade III** TT chirurgical, endoscopique ou radiologique
IIIa sous AL
IIIb sous AG

**Grade IV** complications menaçantes, y compris neurologiques centrales ; indication d'USI ou d'unité de soins intermédiaires
IVa défaillance d'un organe (y compris dialyse)
IVb défaillance multiorganes

**Grade V** DC

Suffixe "d" si le patient présente une complication lors de sa sortie, rajouter "d" (disability) au grade. Ceci indique la nécessité d'un suivi pour évaluation complète de la complication.

**Figure 28** Clavien-Dindo-Strasberg classification (127).

For details of postoperative complications and their gradation, we had used the extension of the Clavien-Dindo classification of surgical complications published by the Japan Clinical Oncology Group (JCOG) in 2016 under the name "Japan Clinical Oncology Group postoperative complications criteria"(128). In this detailed classification, 72 surgical complications had been listed and graded including 17 gastrointestinal, 13 infectious, 6 thoracic and other...

## 9. **Remote monitoring :**

Was done in consultation.

Monitoring schedule and procedures :

- **Clinical examination** every 3 months for 3 years.
- **Abdominal-pelvic ultrasound or Thoraco-abdominal-pelvic CT scan (or alternately)** every 3 to 6 months for 3 years.
- **Colonoscopy** at 3 years (if incomplete pre-operatively, should be scheduled within 6 months post-operatively).
- Quarterly **CEA dosage.**
- **Endorectal ultrasound (EER)** could be proposed in the absence of amputation (transvaginal ultrasound possible in women).
- **Pelvic MRI** if PAA.
- **Hepatic MRI** as a complement to CT if necessary.

### *a) Recidivism:*

After curative surgery, recurrence was detected during surveillance by clinical examination, morphological, endoscopic and/or histological examinations.
Time to recurrence was calculated from the date of initiation of treatment (surgery, chemotherapy or radiotherapy).

### *b) Survival:*

Overall survival and recurrence-free survival were calculated.
The date of origin was the date of initiation of treatment (surgery, chemotherapy or radiotherapy).
The point date has been set for 26/01/2020.

## 10. **Statistical analysis:**

### *a) Statistical tests used :*

Descriptive statistical analysis: frequency, mean, median.

Comparison tests for categorical variables: Chi2 test and Fischer test (for theoretical numbers less than 5) were used.
Test to compare quantitative variables: Student's t-test to compare means.
Survival curves were estimated using the Kaplan-Meier method and compared with the log-rank test.

For multivariate analysis, a Cox regression model including the various covariates of interest was used.

All study values were reported within a 95% confidence interval (the accepted risk of error being 5%), and tests were performed in a two-tailed situation.

Data processing and analysis were carried out using IBM SPSS statistics version 25 software.

### *b) Judging criteria:*

- Judging criteria :
    - Morbidity <30
    - Mortality < 5%.
    - No significant increase in morbidity and mortality compared with the control arm.
    - Conversion rate < 15%.

# VII. Results :

## A. Experimental arm :

Fifty patients who met the inclusion criteria were initially selected.
Four of these patients did not undergo surgery and had been excluded from the study due to progression of their metastatic disease under chemotherapy (Fig.29). Six other patients had undergone laparoscopic surgery but were excluded from the study for various reasons (Fig.30) :

- Discovery of generalized peritoneal carcinosis during laparoscopic exploration in a patient.
- Laparoscopic surgery to remove the primary tumor without approaching the liver in five patients for :
  -Misdiagnosis of liver lesions in two patients (cyst, angioma).
  -Progression of hepatic metastatic disease at the time of surgery in three patients. Of these three patients, only one underwent secondary surgery to remove liver metastases.

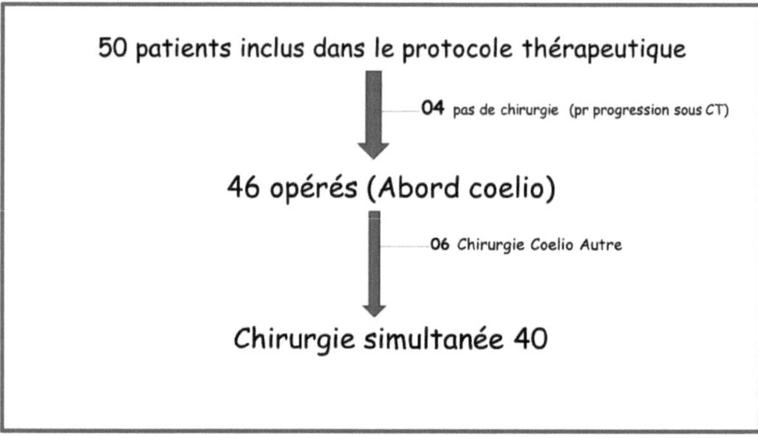


**Figure 29** Inclusion of patients in the study .

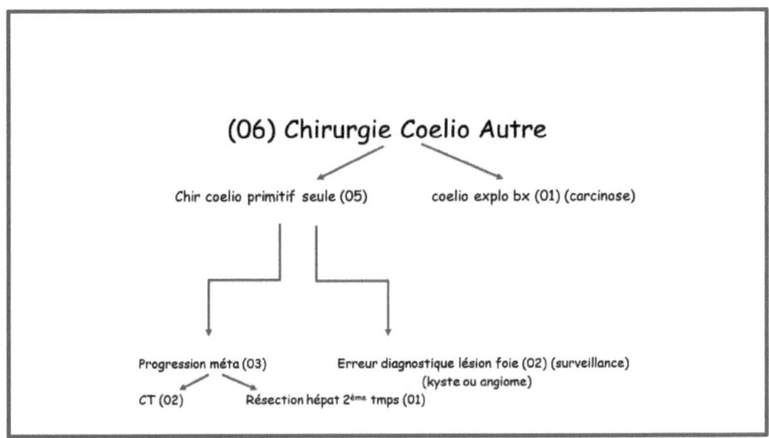


**Figure 30** Excluded surgical patients.

## 1. General patient characteristics:

The number of patients selected for the study (experimental arm) was **40**, distributed as follows:

### *a) Age :*

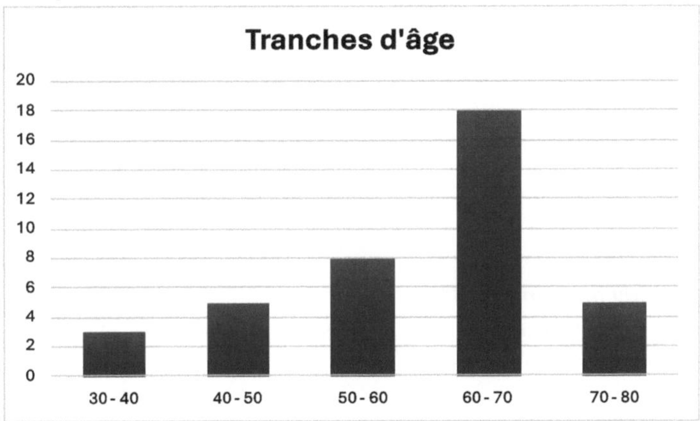


**Figure 31** Histogram of patient distribution by age .

The mean age of patients was 59.08 years, with a median of 62.5 years and extremes of 32 and 79 years.

### *b) Sex:*

We included 23 men and 17 women, for a sex ratio of 1.35.

**Table 9** Distribution of patients by gender.

| Gender | Number | Percentage |
|---|---|---|
| **Men** | 23 | 57,5 % |
| **Women** | 17 | 42,5 % |
| **Total** | 40 | 100 % |

### *c) Distribution of patients by year of inclusion :*

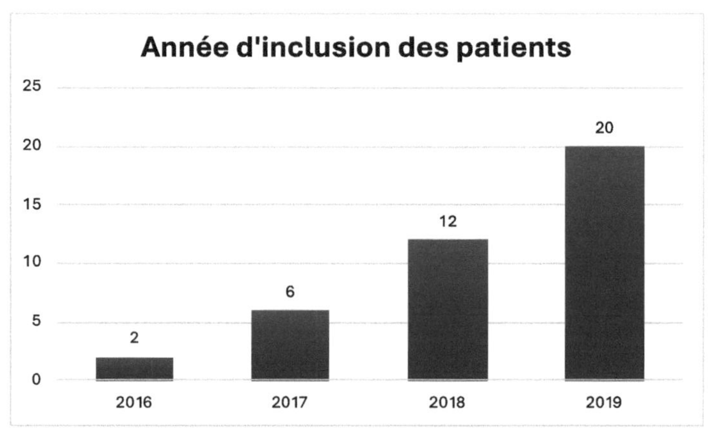


Figure 32 Histogram of patient distribution by year of inclusion.

Thirty-two patients, or 80% of the workforce, had been included in the study during 2018 and 2019.

### *d) Body mass index (BMI) :*

The mean BMI of the patients was 24.05 Kg/m² with a median of 24 Kg/m², the extremes were 18 Kg/m² and 38 Kg/m².

### *e) ASA (American Society of Anesthesiologists):*

The distribution of patients included according to the American Society of Anesthesiologists classification is summarized in Table 10.

**Table 10** Distribution of patients according to ASA classification.

| ASA | Number | Percentage |
|---|---|---|
| **ASA I** | 23 | 57,5 % |

| ASA II | 15 | 37,5 % |
|---|---|---|
| ASA III | 02 | 05,0 % |
| Total | 40 | 100 % |

### *f) Comorbidities:*

Twenty-two patients had comorbidities, i.e. 55% of cases in our series (table 11). Of these, six had more than one comorbidity.

**Table 11** Distribution of patients by comorbidity.

| Comorbidity | Number |
|---|---|
| **Hypertension** | 10 |
| **Diabetes** | 09 |
| **Heart disease** | 03 |
| **Thyroid pathology** | 03 |
| **Other** | 03 |

### *g) WHO performance index :*

All our patients were in good general condition and classified 0 according to the WHO score (performance index) (appendix 6).

### *h) History of abdominal surgery:*

Twelve patients, or 30% of our series, had a history of abdominal surgery (table 12). Of these, three patients had had two previous abdominal surgeries, and one patient had had three.

**Table 12** Summary of abdominal surgery history.

| Pathology/Intervention | Approach | Nb |
|---|---|---|
| **Bulbar ulcer** | Supraumbilical median | 1 |
| **Occlusive colon cancer (colostomy)** | Left iliac elective route | 2 |
| **Occlusive colon cancer (colostomy)** | Median straddling the umbilicus | 2 |
| **Cesarean section** | Pfannenstiel | 3 |
| **Appendectomy** | Mac Burney | 3 |
| **Cholecystectomy** | Laparoscopy | 4 |
| **Nephrectomy** | Lumbotomy | 1 |
| **Foreign body removal** | Xypho-pubic median | 1 |
| **Total** | | 17 |

## 2. Clinical characteristics of patients :

### *a) Telltale symptoms :*

The revealing symptoms that led to the diagnosis are summarized in the following table:

**Table 13** Distribution of revealing symptoms.

| Symptom | Number | Percentage |
|---|---|---|
| **Rectorrhagia** | 12 | 30 % |
| **Rectal syndrome** | 07 | 17,5 % |
| **Transit disorders** | 12 | 30 % |
| **Abdominal pain** | 03 | 7,5 % |
| **Proctalgia** | 02 | 5 % |
| **Anemia** | 04 | 10 % |
| **Total** | 40 | 100 % |

### ***b) Duration of symptoms before consultation :***

**Table 14** Duration of symptoms before consultation in months.

| Duration | ≤ 3 months | 3 to 6 months | > 6 months |
|---|---|---|---|
| **Number** | 16 | 16 | 8 |

### ***c) Location of primary tumor :***

The location was colonic in 60% of cases and rectal in 40% (table 15).

**Table 15** Different locations of the primary tumor.

| Location | Number | Percentage |
|---|---|---|
| **Sigmoid** | 16 | 40 % |
| **Left colon** | 04 | 10 % |
| **Right colon** | 04 | 10 % |
| **Rectum** | 16 | 40 % |
| **Total** | 40 | 100 % |

Rectal locations were distributed as follows (table 16):

**Table 16** Distribution of rectal locations.

| Location | Number | Percentage |
|---|---|---|
| **Upper rectum** | 05 | 31,25 % |
| **Middle rectum** | 06 | 37,50 % |
| **Lower rectum** | 05 | 31,25 % |
| **Total** | 16 | 100 % |

### ***d) Biopsy:***

Endoscopic biopsy of the primary tumor for diagnostic purposes had revealed the following histological findings:

**Table 17** Histological results of biopsy.

| Biopsy | Number | Percentage |
|---|---|---|
| **Well-differentiated adenocarcinoma** | 29 | 72,5 % |
| **Moderately differentiated adenocarcinoma** | 10 | 25,0 % |
| **Independent cell mucosecretory carcinoma** | 01 | 2,5 % |
| **Total** | 40 | 100 % |

RAS status was determined from biopsies in 19 patients, with mutation present in 12.

### *e) Metastasis:*

#### (1) Location:

Liver metastases were unilobar in 72.5% of patients (Table 18), with segments VI and VII the most frequently affected (Table 19).

**Table 18** Hepatic location of metastases.

| Location | Number | Percentage |
|---|---|---|
| **Unilobar** | 29 | 72,5 % |
| **Bilobar** | 11 | 27,5 % |
| **Total** | 40 | 100 % |

**Table 19** Liver segments affected by metastases.

| Segments | Patient |
|---|---|
| **I** | 00 |
| **II** | 06 |
| **III** | 10 |
| **IV a** | 06 |
| **IV b** | 08 |
| **V** | 10 |
| **VI** | 22 |
| **VII** | 23 |
| **VIII** | 12 |

#### (2) The number :

Seventeen patients had a single metastasis; in patients with multiple metastases, the number ranged from 02 to 11 metastases.

**Table 20** Distribution of metastases according to whether they are single or multiple.

| Number | Patient | Percentage |
|---|---|---|
| **Unique** | 17 | 42,5 % |
| **Multiple** | 23 | 57,5 % |
| **Total** | 40 | 100 % |

**Table 21** Distribution by number of metastases.

| Number | Patient | Percentage |
|---|---|---|
| **01** | 17 | 42,5 % |
| **02** | 08 | 20,0 % |
| **03** | 02 | 05,0 % |
| > **03** | 13 | 32,5 % |
| **Total** | 40 | 100 % |

### (3) Size:

The size of the largest liver metastasis per patient averaged 39.95 mm, with a median of 39 mm. Extreme sizes were 6 mm and 88 mm.

## 3. Pre-therapeutic classification :

After the clinical and paraclinical extension workup, patients were classified according to the c TNM classification as follows:

**Table 22** Distribution of patients according to TNM c classification.

| cTNM class | Number | Percentage |
|---|---|---|
| **T2N0M1a** | 02 | 5,0 % |
| **T2N+M1a** | 01 | 2,5 % |
| **T3N0M1a** | 03 | 7,5 % |
| **T3N+M1a** | 34 | 85 % |
| **Total** | 40 | 100 % |

The majority of patients were classified as cT3N+M1a.

## 4. Neoadjuvant treatment :

Thirty-four patients (85% of cases) had received neoadjuvant treatment, either perioperative chemotherapy, neoadjuvant drug therapy (chemotherapy plus targeted therapy), short radiotherapy or concomitant radiochemotherapy (CCT). These therapies could be combined in the case of a rectal primary. Several treatment sequences were possible (Table 23):

**Table 23** Summary of neoadjuvant treatment modalities.

| Therapeutic sequence | Number | Percentage |
|---|---|---|
| **CT+TC then surgery** | 17 | 50,00 % |
| **Perioperative CT followed by surgery** | 07 | 20,59 % |
| **CT then short RT then immediate surgery** | 03 | 08,82 % |
| **Short RT followed by immediate surgery** | 02 | 08,82 % |
| **CCR then delayed surgery** | 02 | 08,82 % |
| **CT+TC then short RT then deferred surgery** | 01 | 02,94 % |
| **CT then short RT then deferred surgery** | 01 | 02,94 % |
| **Short RT followed by delayed surgery** | 01 | 02,94 % |
| **Total** | 34 | 100 % |

### *a) Radiotherapy:*

Radiotherapy was administered to 10 patients (25% of cases) with metastatic tumors of the lower or middle rectum classified as T3 or N+.

Two radiotherapy protocols were used:

Most patients (80%) opted for the short protocol, which administered a 25Gy dose fractionated over 5 days.

In 2 patients (20%), concomitant radiochemotherapy of the CAP 50 type was administered, combining 50 Gy in 25 fractions spread over 5 weeks (2 Gy per fraction) with concomitant chemotherapy: capecitabine (1,600 mg/m2 divided into 1 morning and evening dose of 800 mg/m2 on radiotherapy days).

**Table 24** The radiosurgical sequence.

| Surgical X-ray sequence | Number | Percentage |
|---|---|---|
| **RT short immediate surgery** | 05 | 50% |
| **Delayed surgery short RT** | 03 | 30% |
| **RCC deferred surgery** | 02 | 20% |
| **Total** | 10 | 100 % |

### *b) Chemotherapy / Targeted therapy :*

Twenty-nine patients (72.5% of cases) had received preoperative chemotherapy with or without targeted therapy to control metastatic disease.

Chemotherapy was administered either alone perioperatively in the case of resectable liver metastases, or in combination with targeted therapy in the case of potentially resectable liver metastases.

Targeted therapy could be an anti-angiogenic antibody (Bevacizumab) or an anti-EGFR (Cetuximab or Panitumumab), with the choice depending on RAS status (wild-type or mutated).

The different protocols used in our series were as follows:

**Table 25** Chemotherapy protocols used.

| Protocol | Number | Percentage |
|---|---|---|
| **FOLFOX** | 10 | 34,48 % |
| **CAPOX** | 01 | 03,45 % |
| **CAPOX + Bevacizumab** | 03 | 10,34 % |
| **CAPOX + Cetuximab** | 02 | 06,90 % |
| **FOLFOX + Panitumumab** | 02 | 06,90 % |
| **CAPOX + Panitumumab** | 01 | 03,45 % |
| **FOLFOX + Bevacizumab** | 08 | 27,59 % |
| **FOLFOX + Cetuximab** | 02 | 06,89 % |
| **Total** | 29 | 100 % |

The number of preoperative cures averaged 5.97, with a median of 6 and extremes of 3 to 13.
The interval between the last course of chemotherapy and surgery averaged 6.31 weeks, with a median of 5 weeks, and the extremes were 3 and 12 weeks respectively.

### c) *Response to neoadjuvant treatment :*

#### (1) Response to radiotherapy:

The response of the primary rectal tumor to radiotherapy was assessed by pelvic MRI at 4 weeks when surgery was deferred.
Delayed surgery concerned 5 patients, 2 after RCC and 3 after short RT.
Re-evaluation was carried out in 4 patients, each time showing a partial reduction in rectal parietal thickening.
One patient had not been reassessed after short RT.

#### (2) Response to drug treatment :

The response of metastatic disease to drug treatment, whether chemotherapy alone or chemotherapy combined with targeted therapy, was assessed radiologically by TAP CT according to RECIST 1.1 criteria (Response Evaluation Criteria in Solid Tumors).
Twenty-nine patients had received preoperative chemotherapy with or without targeted therapy. The results of the reassessment are summarized in the following table:

**Table 26** Evaluation of drug therapy according to RECIST.

| RECIST | Number | Percentage |
|---|---|---|
| **Progression** | 00 | 00 % |
| **Stability** | 17 | 58,62 % |
| **Partial response** | 12 | 41,38 % |

| Full answer | 00 | 00 % |
|---|---|---|
| Total | 29 | 100 % |

The objective response (OR) represents the sum of partial responses and complete responses (OR = CR + PR) **(OR = 41.38%).**
Tumor control (TC) is the sum of complete responses, partial responses and stable disease (TC=CR+PR+MS) **(TC = 100%).**

## 5. Surgery features :

### *a) Strategy:*

The two tumor sites, primary colorectal and secondary hepatic, were approached using three different modalities; the distribution of patients according to these 3 modalities is summarized in Table 27 :

**Table 27** Surgical management procedures

| Modality | Number | Percentage |
|---|---|---|
| **All laparoscopic** | 04 | 10 % |
| **Hybrid surgery** | 24 | 60 % |
| **"down staging" surgery** | 09 | 22,5 % |
| **Conversion** | 03 | 7,5 % |
| **Total** | 40 | 100% |

### *b) All laparoscopic:*

Four patients representing 10% of the total series had a pure laparoscopic approach to curatively resect both tumor sites, the colorectal primary and liver metastases during the same surgical procedure.

### (1) Trocar arrangement/Extraction incision:

After the exploration phase, the surgical procedure began with the colorectal resection phase. For this, the trocars were arranged in the standard way, with five trocars in place, an 11 mm umbilical optical trocar, and four operating trocars (12 mm trocar in the right iliac fossa, 05 mm trocar on the left flank, 05 mm trocar on the right hypochondrium, and a fifth 5 or 10 mm trocar in the suprapubic position).

After the colorectal resection, the anastomosis was deferred. The liver resection was performed first, after the addition of a 5mm epigastric trocar.

Once the liver had been resected, the surgical specimens (colorectal and liver) were extracted through a Pfannenstiel incision.
Anastomosis was then performed.

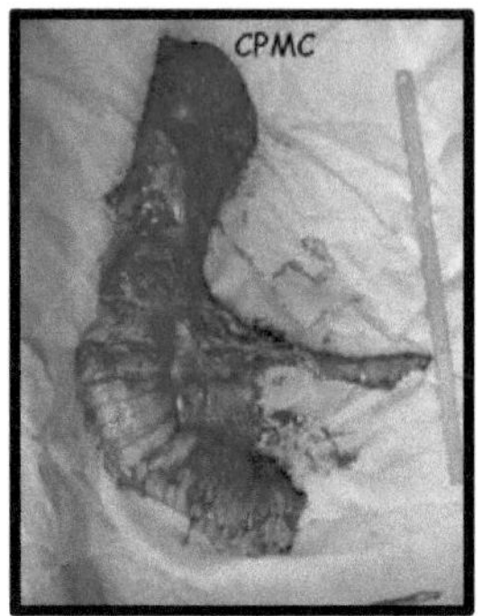


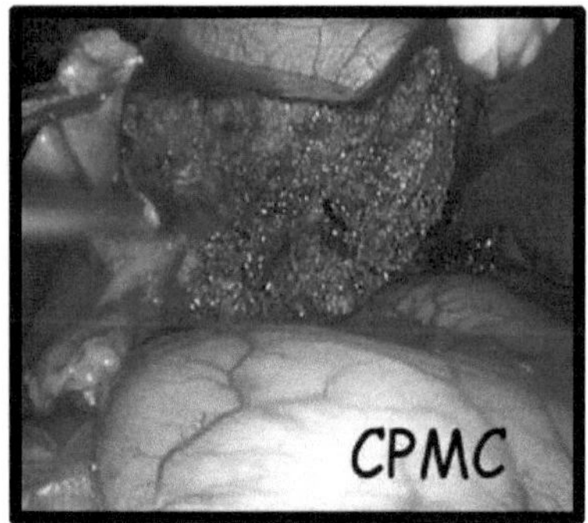


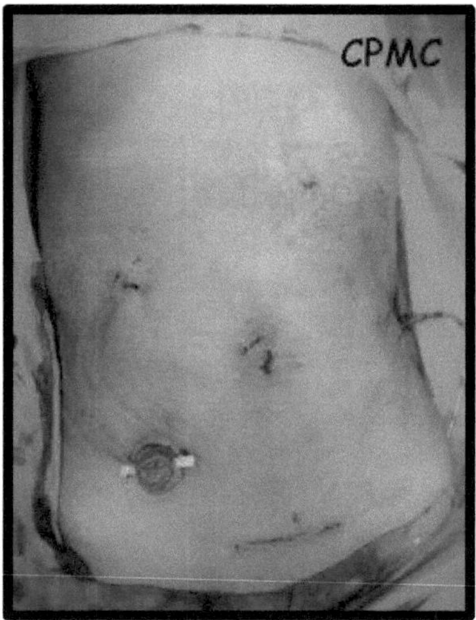


**Figure 33** Totally laparoscopic surgery for rectal tumor with segment III liver metastasis (CPMC).

## (2) The surgical procedure :

The surgical procedures performed during laparoscopic surgery are summarized in the following table:

**Table 28** Details of surgical procedures in the case of so-called ″tout laparoscopic″ surgery.

| Primi | Metastasis | Incision | Laparoscopic liver surgery | Operating time in minutes | Intraoperative | Clamping | Drainage |
|---|---|---|---|---|---|---|---|

| | tive | (segment) | Laparoscopic colorectal surgery | | | Primitive | Metastasis | ultrasound | | Colorectal | Liver |
|---|---|---|---|---|---|---|---|---|---|---|---|
| **01** | Lower rectum | III | RA+ETM+ACA+ileostomy | Pfannenstiel | Wedge resection III | 290 | 90 | - | - | + | - |
| **02** | Upper rectum | III | RA+EPM+ACR | Pfannenstiel | Wedge resection III | 260 | 40 | - | - | + | - |
| **03** | Middle rectum | III, IVa | RA+ETM+ACSA+ileostomy | Pfannenstiel | Double metastasectomy III, IVa | 270 | 90 | - | - | + | - |
| **04** | Middle rectum | III | RA+ETM+ACSA+ileostomy+right annexectomy | Pfannenstiel | Metastasectomy III | 260 | 50 | - | - | + | - |

### *c) Hybrid surgery:*

Twenty-four patients, representing 60% of the total series, had a mixed laparoscopic and laparotomic approach, with the aim of achieving complete curative resection of the primary tumor and liver metastases simultaneously.

### (1) Approach :

The laparoscopic approach to colorectal tumors was performed with 4 trocars in the case of a colonic primary, or with 5 trocars in the case of a rectal primary (table 29) :

**Table 29** Number of trocars used.

| Number of trocars | Patients | Percentage |
|---|---|---|
| **04** | 14 | 58,33 % |
| **05** | 10 | 41,67 % |
| **Total** | 24 | 100 % |

Liver metastases were approached via a median supraumbilical incision, a right subcutaneous incision or a Makuuchi incision.
The choice of incision type depended on the location of liver metastases.
This incision was also often used to extract the surgical specimen or prepare the colonic transplant for anastomosis (table 30).

**Table 30** Incision types in hybrid surgery.

| Type of incision | Patient | Percentage |
|---|---|---|
| **Umbilical median** | 01 | 04,17 % |
| **Right subcostal** | 04 | 16,67 % |
| **Makuuchi incision** | 19 | 79,16 % |
| **Total** | 24 | 100 % |

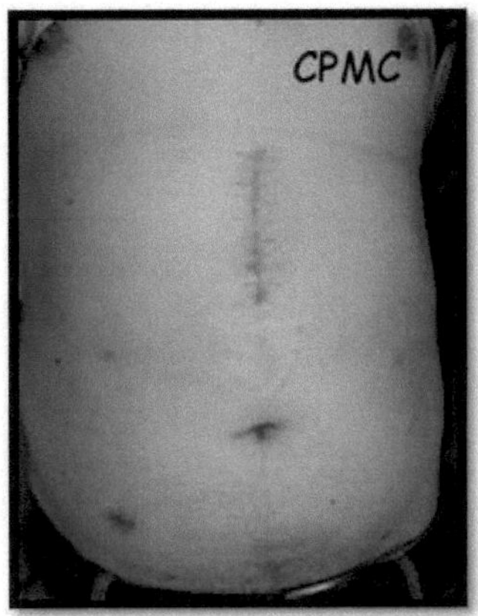


**Figure 34** Hybrid surgery using a median supraumbilical incision (CPMC).

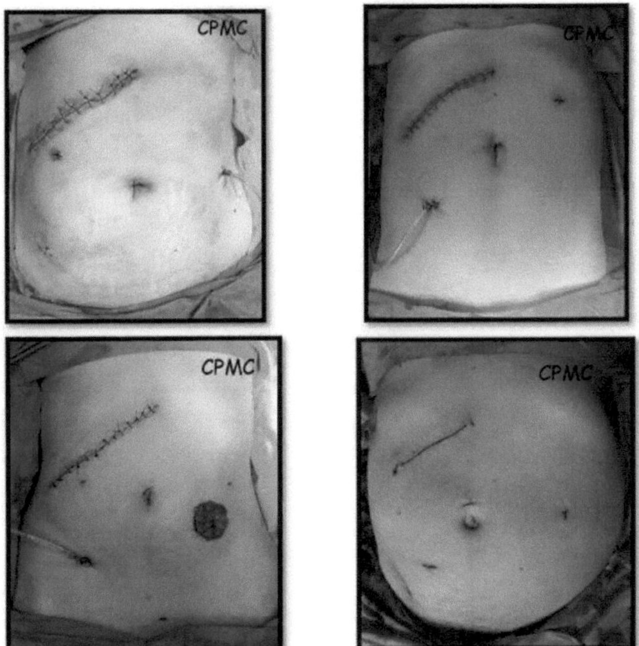


**Figure 35** Hybrid surgery using a right subcostal incision (RSCI).

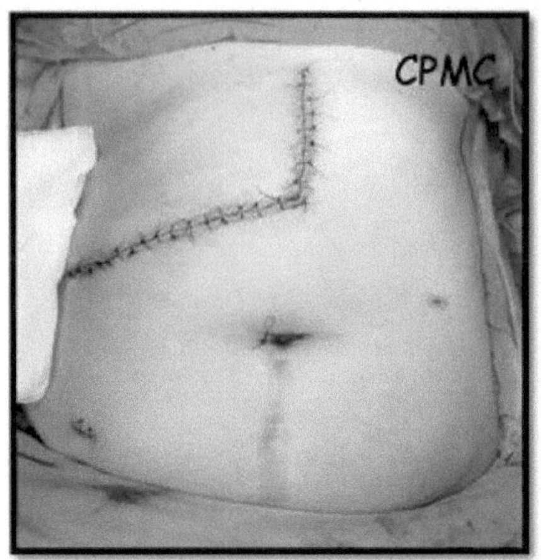


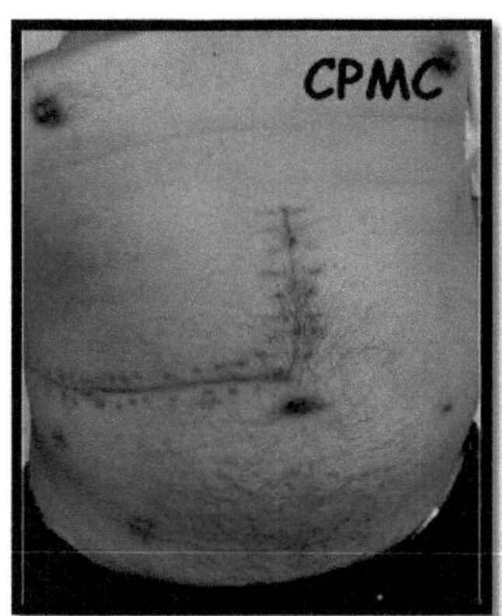


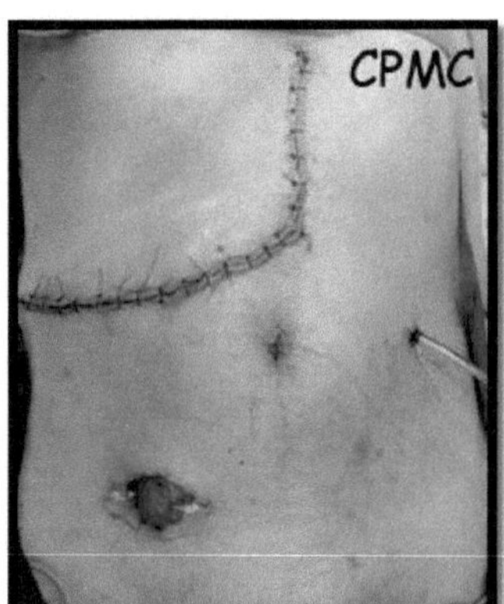


**Figure 36** Hybrid surgery using a Makuuchi incision (CPMC).

## (2) The surgical procedure :

The surgical procedures performed during hybrid surgery are summarized in the following table:

**Table 31** Details of surgical procedures for hybrid surgery.

| | Primitive | Metastasis | Laparoscopic procedure | Incision | Laparotomy procedure | Operating time in minutes | | Echographie | Clamping | Drainage | |
|---|---|---|---|---|---|---|---|---|---|---|---|
| | | | | | | Primitive | Metastasis | | | Colorectal | Liver |
| 01 | Sigmoid | VI,VII | Low segment resection | Makuuchi | Double metastasectomy VI, VII | 270 | 60 | - | - | + | + |
| 02 | Left colon | III | Left colonic resection | Median | Wedge resection III | 265 | 90 | - | - | + | - |
| 03 | Upper rectum | VII | RA+EPM+ACR | Makuuchi | Wedge resection VII | 235 | 55 | - | - | + | - |
| 04 | Middle rectum | IVb | RA+ETM+ACSA+ileostomy | Makuuchi | Segmentectomy IVb | 270 | 90 | + | + | + | - |
| 05 | Left colon | III,IVa,IVb,VI, VII | Left colonic resection | Makuuchi | Metastasectomy III, segmentectomy IV, subsegmentectomy VI, subsegmentectomy VII | 220 | 200 | + | + | - | + |
| 06 | Sigmoid | IVb, VI | Low segmental resection, including stoma | Makuuchi | Segmentectomy IVb, wedge resection VI | 150 | 150 | - | - | - | - |
| 07 | Right colon | VI, VII | Right hemicolectomy | Makuuchi | Sub-segmentectomy VI, sub-segmentectomy VII | 150 | 150 | + | + | - | + |
| 08 | Lower rectum | VII | AAP | Makuuchi | Metastasectomy VII | 300 | 90 | - | + | + | - |
| 09 | Right colon | VII | Right hemicolectomy | Makuuchi | Segmentectomy VII | 150 | 150 | - | + | - | + |
| 10 | Left colon | IVb, V, VI | Left colonic resection | Makuuchi | Wedge resection straddling IVb,V,VI | 220 | 120 | - | + | - | - |
| 11 | Middle rectum | VI, VII | RA+ETM+ACSA+ileostomy | Makuuchi | Sub-segmentectomy VI, metastasectomy VII | 240 | 90 | - | - | + | - |
| 12 | Sigmoid | VI | Low segmental resection extended to the right adnexa | Subcostal | Wedge resection VI | 240 | 90 | + | - | + | - |
| 13 | Sigmoid | VI,VII | Low segment resection | Makuuchi | VI segmentectomy extended to VII | 240 | 150 | - | + | + | - |
| 14 | Right colon | VI,VII | Right hemicolectomy | Makuuchi | Sub-segmentectomy VII, double metastasectomy VII, scar resection VI | 180 | 180 | - | - | - | + |
| 15 | Sigmoid | IVa, VIII | Low segment resection | Makuuchi | Double metastasectomy IVa, VIII | 150 | 120 | - | - | - | - |
| 16 | Lower rectum | IVb | AAP | Subcostal | Segmentectomy IVb | 180 | 150 | - | - | + | - |
| 17 | Sigmoid | VIII | Low segment resection | Subcostal | Ultrasound for radiofrequency treatment | 200 | 20 | + | - | - | - |
| 18 | Middle rectum | VI, VII | RA+ETM+ACSA+ileostomy | Subcostal | Sub-segmentectomy VI, metastasectomy VII | 300 | 120 | + | - | + | - |

| 19 | Upper rectum | VI,VII | RA+ACR | Makuuchi | Posterior sectorectomy | 195 | 165 | - | + | - | + |
|---|---|---|---|---|---|---|---|---|---|---|---|
| 20 | Lower rectum | V, VIII | RA+ETM+ACA+ileostomy | Makuuchi | Exploration, liver staging | 270 | 30 | - | - | + | - |
| 21 | Upper rectum | VI, VII | Left colorectal resection enlarged to the right + Deloyer | Makuuchi | Double metastasectomy VI, Wedge resection VII | 300 | 120 | - | + | - | + |
| 22 | Sigmoid | VI,VII | Left colonic resection with stoma removed | Makuuchi | Wedge resection VI, VII | 270 | 90 | - | + | - | + |
| 23 | Lower rectum | VI,VII | RA+ETM+ACA+ileostomy | Makuuchi | Wedge resection VI,VII | 240 | 120 | - | - | + | - |
| 24 | Sigmoid | V,VI | Low segmental resection extended to the left adnexa | Makuuchi | Wedge straddle resection V,VI | 180 | 120 | - | + | - | - |

### *d) Laparoscopic "down staging" surgery:*

Nine patients, i.e. 22.5% of the total series, had undergone laparoscopic first-stage hepatectomy for multiple bilobar metastases:

- 6 patients underwent laparoscopic resection of the primary tumour + laparoscopic portal ligation +/- laparoscopic surgery of liver metastases on one hemi-loin followed, a few weeks later, by a major hepatectomy via the conventional route.

- 3 patients underwent a first hybrid resection ( laparoscopic resection of the primary tumour combined with resection of part of the liver metastases), followed in a second phase (deferred by a few weeks) by surgery to remove the rest of the liver metastases by conventional means.

### (1) Arrangement of trocars / Incisions :

In the first approach for the 6 patients, the trocar layout followed that of the "tout laparoscopique", with the epigastric trocar added for the hepatic step, in addition to the 4 or 5 trocars used for the colorectal step (4 for the colon, 5 for the rectum). The incision used to extract the surgical parts was a Pfannenstiel incision in 5 patients.
One patient in this group had a laparoscopic liver section, followed by a colorectal section performed partly laparoscopically and completed by a median approach, since a Deloyer-type colonic lowering maneuver was required in this patient. This route was also used to extract the parts.

In the second approach for the remaining 3 patients, the trocar arrangement was the same for the colorectal stage (4 trocars), followed by a median supraumbilical incision in 2 patients, or Makuuchi in one patient for the liver stage, which consisted of resection of the most accessible liver metastases (minor resection). A second, complementary hepatic stage was required after a few weeks, with the aim of achieving complete R0 resection.

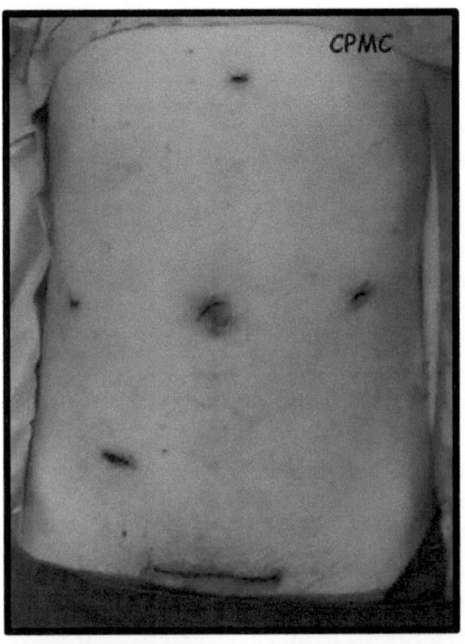


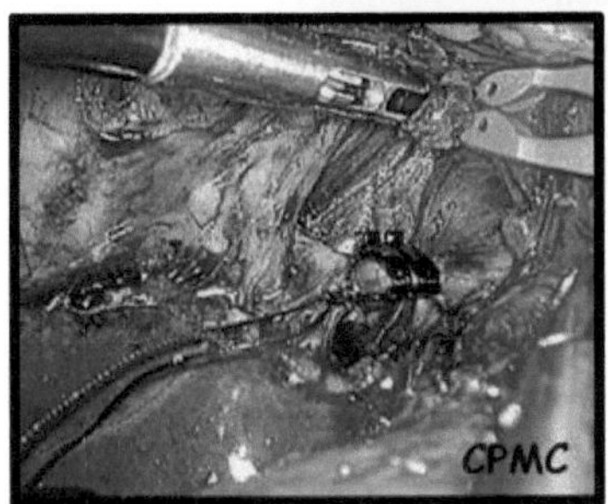


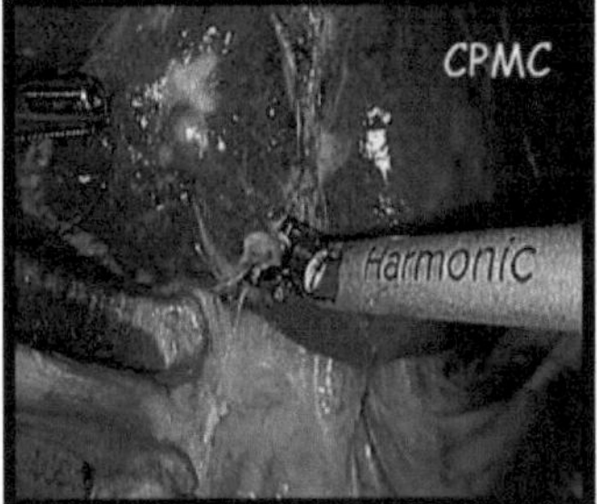


**Figure 37** Laparoscopic "Down staging" surgery with right portal ligation (CPMC ).

## (2) The surgical procedure :

The surgical procedures performed during "down staging" surgery are summarized in the following table:

**Table 32** Details of surgical procedures for "down staging" surgery with portal ligation.

| | Primitive | Metastasis | Laparoscopic colorectal surgery | Incision | Laparoscopic liver surgery | Operating time in minutes | | Ultrasound | Clamping | Drainage | |
|---|---|---|---|---|---|---|---|---|---|---|---|
| | | | | | | Primitive | Metastasis | | | Colorectal | Liver |
| 01 | Sigmoid | II,III,VI,VII,VIII | Low segment resection | Pfannenstiel | Metastasectomy II, right portal ligation | 165 | 100 | - | - | - | - |
| 02 | Sigmoid | II,IV,V,VIII | Low segmental resection, resection, including stoma | Stomial | Left portal ligature | 270 | 90 | - | - | - | - |
| 03 | Left colon | VI,VII, VIII | Left colectomy | Pfannenstiel | Right portal ligature | 255 | 45 | - | - | - | - |
| 04 | Sigmoid | VI,VII, VIII | Low segment resection | Pfannenstiel | Right portal ligature | 180 | 80 | - | - | - | - |
| 05 | Sigmoid | II,III,V,VIII | Low segment resection | Pfannenstiel | Wedge resection III, right portal ligation | 210 | 90 | - | - | - | - |
| 06 | Sigmoid | III,V,VI,VII | Left colonic resection enlarged to the right with stoma + Deloyer | Median | Metastasectomy III, right portal ligation | 150 | 155 | - | - | - | - |

**Table 33** Details of surgical procedures for ″down staging″ surgery without portal ligation.

| | Primitive | Metastasis | Laparoscopic colorectal surgery | Incision | Hepatic surgery by laparotomy | Operating time in minutes | | Ultrasound | Clamping | Drainage | |
|---|---|---|---|---|---|---|---|---|---|---|---|
| | | | | | | Primitive | Metastasis | | | Colorectal | Liver |
| 07 | Sigmoid | III, IVa,VII,VIII | Low segment resection | Median | Wedge resection III | 165 | 45 | - | - | + | - |
| 08 | Upper rectum | II,III,IVb, V,VI,VII, VIII | RA+EPM +ACR | Median | Wedge resection III + Metastasectomy IV b+ | 195 | 60 | - | - | - | - |

|  |  |  |  |  | Metastasectomy II-III |  |  |  |  |  |  |
|---|---|---|---|---|---|---|---|---|---|---|---|
| **09** | Sigmoid | II,IVa,IVb,V,VI,VII,VIII | Low segment resection | Makuuchi | Wedge resection II, IVb metastasectomy VIII,wedge VI-VII | 188 | 182 | + | - | - | + |

## e) *Conversion :*

We considered **conversion** to be the necessity of performing the entire surgical procedure (colorectal and liver times) by laparotomy.

Strictly speaking, we had to convert three patients, corresponding to a conversion rate of 7.5%. The causes of conversion were :

Case 1: 79-year-old patient, ASA I, no previous history, with adenocarcinoma of the middle rectum associated with a single liver metastasis straddling segments V and VI. Had received neoadjuvant CCR.

Trocar placement was impossible due to the highly adherent nature of the abdominal cavity and intestinal loops (probable infectious sequelae) (Fig.38).

Conversion was decided at the beginning of the operation via a median xypho-pubic approach.

The procedure performed was an anterior resection with total removal of the mesorectum and mechanical latero-terminal colo-sus-anal anastomosis associated with a wedge resection straddling segments V and VI.

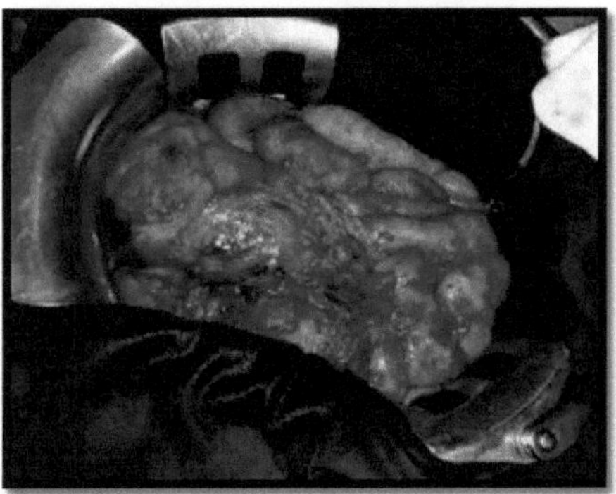

**Figure 38** Aspect of handles after conversion case n°1 (CPMC).

Case 2: ASAII patient, 72 years old, diabetic, with the following surgical history: right subcostal cholecystectomy, total thyroidectomy complicated by chronic hypoparathyroidism, two median subumbilical caesarean sections. Her BMI was 30 kg/m².

She presented with adenocarcinoma of the right colon associated with a single liver metastasis straddling segments V and VI.
A 4-trocar laparoscopic approach was performed, and after freeing a few adhesions, a primary approach to the right colonic vessels was undertaken. The patient then developed hemodynamic problems, forcing us to reduce insufflation pressures from 12 mm Hg to 10 mm Hg and then to 8 mm Hg. Despite this, the problems persisted and worsened with the onset of tachycardia. By mutual agreement with the anesthesia and intensive care team, the decision was taken to convert the patient. The procedure (double resection) was completed by Makuuchi laparotomy. A right hemicolectomy with terminal-lateral ileo-transverse anastomosis and a wedge resection straddling segments V and VI were performed (Fig.39).

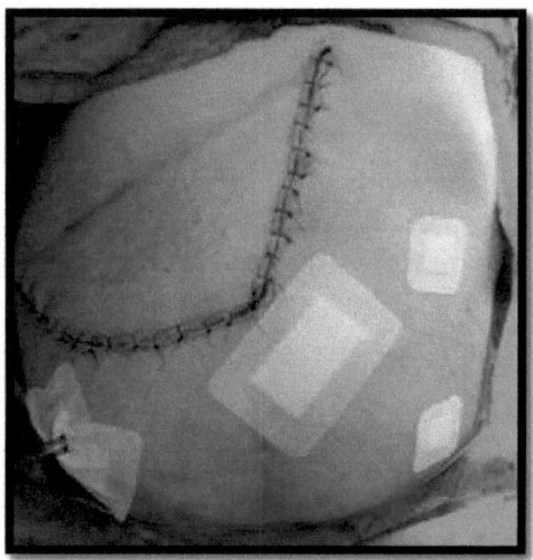

**Figure 39** Conversion for intolerance of pneumoperitoneum, case 2 (CPMC).

Case 3: 65-year-old patient, ASA I, with no previous history, presenting with a double colonic tumour location (sigmoid and right colic), associated with two hepatic metastases of segments VII and VIII classified cT3N+M1a.
A laparoscopic approach revealed a T4 tumor infiltrating the anterior wall, bladder and ileal loop, associated with localized carcinosis.
The conversion was decided in view of these findings.
Approached via a median xypho-pubic incision, the procedure performed was a total colectomy enlarged to include a bladder lozenge, ileal loop and anterior parietal lozenge, combined with douglassectomy and double metastasectomy VII, VIII (Fig.40).

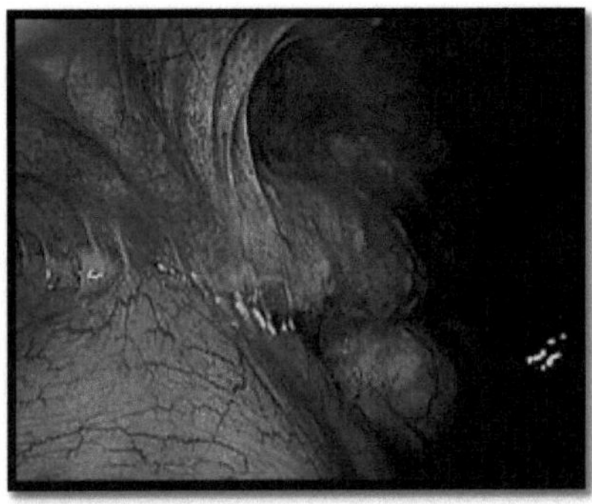

**Figure 40** Laparoscopic finding of T4 tumor, localized carcinosis. Case 3 (CPMC).

| | *p* value |
|---|---|
| **ASA** | 0,894 |
| **BMI** | 0,615 |
| **Previous abdominal surgery** | 0,704 |
| **Previous median incision** | 0,338 |
| **Intraoperative incidents (Oslo)** | **0,044** |
| **pT(TNM)** | **0,011** |

**Table 34** Conversion risk factors.

After statistical analysis (table 34), two factors were associated with the occurrence of a conversion: the degree of severity of the intraoperative incident according to the grades of the Oslo classification, and the degree of parietal infiltration on anatomopathological study.

### *f) Exploratory laparoscopy :*

The diagnostic role of laparoscopy enabled us to correct our attitude in two patients:

- One patient was secondarily excluded from the study, as laparoscopy had revealed generalized peritoneal carcinosis that had not been suspected during the initial clinical and morphological extension work-up.

Intracelioscopic biopsies had been performed, confirming carcinosis.

This diagnostic laparoscopy avoided an unnecessary laparotomy.

The patient had been referred to medical oncology for initiation of drug therapy, the primary tumor was nonsymptomatic.

- A previously described patient (case 3) with a T4 tumor requiring conversion. Here too, laparoscopy was superior to the initial extension work-up.

### g) *Pedicle clamping :*

Hepatic clamping was not systematically performed, because of the risk to the digestive anastomosis, and several modalities were possible: selective clamping, pedicle clamping (intermittent clamping or continuous clamping).
Intermittent clamping consisted of clamping for 10 to 15 min then declamping for 05 min then reclamping if necessary for 10 to 15 min.
Clamping was performed in 12 patients (30% of the total), with pedicle clamping in 10 and selective clamping in 2.
The various hepatic clamping procedures are summarized in Table 35.

| Clamping | YES | | NO |
|---|---|---|---|
| | 12 (30%) | | 28 (70%) |
| | Type | Pedicular 10 | |
| | | Selective 02 | |
| | Average pedicle clamping time: 14.5 mn (8mn-30mn) | | |

**Table 35** Hepatic clamping procedures.

| | Primitive | Metastasis | Colorectal gesture | Hepatic gesture | Clamping type | Clamping time in minutes |
|---|---|---|---|---|---|---|
| 01 | Middle rectum | IVb | RA+ETM+ACSA+ileostomy | Segmentectomy IVb | Pedicular | 08 mn |
| 02 | Left colon | III,IVa,IVb, VI, VII | Left colonic resection | Metastasectomy III, segmentectectomy IV, subsegmentectomy VI, subsegmentectomy VII | Selective right / Selective left | Left 15 min, right 8 min, left 15 min, right 10 min and right 13 min |
| 03 | Right colon | VI, VII | Right hemicolectomy | Sub-segment VI, sub-segment VII | Pedicular | 19 mn |
| 04 | Lower rectum | VII | AAP | Metastasectomy VII | Pedicular | 10 mn |
| 05 | Right colon | VII | Right hemicolectomy | Segmentectomy VII | Pedicular | 15 mn |

| 06 | Left colon | IVb, V, VI | Left colonic resection | Wedge resection straddling IVb,V,VI | Pedicular | 15 mn |
|---|---|---|---|---|---|---|
| 07 | Sigmoid | VI,VII | Low segment resection | VI segmentectomy extended to VII | Pedicular | 17 mn then 13 mn |
| 08 | Upper rectum | VI,VII | RA+ACR | Posterior sectorectomy | Right-hand selective | 19 mn |
| 09 | Upper rectum | VI, VII | Left colorectal resection enlarged to the right + Deloyer | Double metastasectomy VI, Wedge resection VII | Pedicular | 10 min then 4 min |
| 10 | Sigmoid | VI,VII | Left colonic resection with stoma removed | Wedge resection VI, VII | Pedicular | 14 mn |
| 11 | Middle rectum | V,VI | RA+ETM+ACSA+ileostomy | Wedge straddle resection V,VI | Pedicular | 10 mn |
| 12 | Sigmoid | V,VI | Low segmental resection extended to the left adnexa | Wedge straddle resection V,VI | Pedicular | 10 mn |

**Table 36** Type and duration of clamping per patient.

## *h) Intraoperative ultrasound :*

Intraoperative ultrasonography was not systematically performed in 7 patients (17.5% of the entire series).

**Table 37** Intraoperative ultrasound goals per patient.

| | Primitive | Metastasis | Laparoscopic procedure | Laparotomy procedure | Ultrasound | Goal |
|---|---|---|---|---|---|---|
| 01 | Middle rectum | Deep IVb in contact with portal pedicle | RA+ETM+ACSA+ileostomy | Segmentectomy IVb | + | Detection/ reporting |
| 02 | Left colon | III,IVa,IVb,VI, VII deep multiple | Left colonic resection | Metastasectomy III, segmentectomy IV, subsegmentectomy VI, subsegmentectomy VII | + | Detection |
| 03 | Right colon | VI, VII deep | Right hemicolectomy | Sub-segmentectomy VI, sub-segmentectomy VII | + | Detection |
| 04 | Sigmoid | Deep sub-centimetric VI | Lower segment resection extended to the right adnexa | Wedge resection VI | + | Detection |
| 05 | Sigmoid | VIII deep | Low-segment resection | Ultrasound for radiofrequency treatment | + | Detection |
| 06 | Middle rectum | VI, VII deep | RA+ETM+ACSA+ileostomy | Sub-segmentectomy VI, metastasectomy VII | + | Detection |
| 07 | Sigmoid | II,IVa,IVb,V,VI,VII,VIII multiple | Low segment resection | Wedge resection II, IV b, metastasectomy VIII, wedge VI-VII | + | Detection, exploration |

## *i) Drainage:*

Drainage was not systematic; 28 patients (70% of the total) had been drained. The two drainage sites (colorectal resection site, hepatic resection site) were drained differently (table 38):

**Table 38** Types of abdominal drainage in patients.

| Drainage | YES | NO |
|---|---|---|

| | 28 (70 %) | | 12 (30 %) |
|---|---|---|---|
| | Type | Colorectal site only 20 | |
| | | Liver site only 07 | |
| | | Two 01 sites | |

### j) *Operating time :*

The average operating time for our series was 323 min for the total duration of the procedure. 221.8 min for colorectal time and 101.2 min for liver time.
Average operating times by type of procedure are summarized in the following table:

**Table 39** Average operating times by type of procedure.

| | Primitive | Liver | Total | *p* value |
|---|---|---|---|---|
| All laparoscopic | 270 mn | 67.5 mn | 337.5 mn | 0,568 |
| Hybrid Surgery | 225 mn | 113 mn | 338 mn | **0,017** |
| Down staging surgery +/- portal ligation | 197.5 mn | 94.1 mn | 291.6 mn | **0,041** |
| Conversion | 200 mn | 70 mn | 270 mn | 0,069 |
| Average operating time in series | 221.8 mn | 101.2 mn | 323 mn | |

Operating time for hybrid surgery was longer than for other procedures ($p$ = 0.017).
The duration of down-staging surgery was the shortest among the different procedures ($p$ = 0.041).

### k) *Postoperative pain:*

Assessed at 24$^{ème}$ hours using a visual analog scale, the results were as follows:

**Table 40** Postoperative pain according to a visual analog scale VAS.

| Pain | 1/10 | 2/10 | 3/10 | 4/10 | 5/10 | 6/10 | 7/10 | 8/10 | 9/10 | 10/10 |
|---|---|---|---|---|---|---|---|---|---|---|
| Number | 07 | 18 | 09 | 04 | 01 | 01 | - | - | - | - |

## l) *Resuming transit :*

**Table 41** Transit resumption time in days.

| Resuming transit | J01 | J02 | J03 | J04 | J05 |
|---|---|---|---|---|---|
| Number | 16 | 19 | 04 | 01 | - |

## m) *Two-stage hepatectomies:*

Nine patients (22.5% of the total) with multiple bilobar liver metastases required a two-stage hepatectomy to achieve curative resection of all metastases.

Six patients had insufficient liver volume on volumetry and required portal ligation during the first laparoscopic stage.

The following tables summarize volumes before and after portal ligation, as well as re-operation times and type of hepatectomy.

**Table 42** Two-stage hepatectomies after portal ligation.

| | Primitive | Metastasis | First intervention | Second intervention | Third intervention |
|---|---|---|---|---|---|
| **01** | Sigmoid | II,III,VI,VII, VIII | Low segmental resection, Metastasectomy II, right portal ligation | 1er ALPPS time | 2ème ALPPS time (right hepatectomy) |
| **02** | Sigmoid | II,IV,V,VIII | Low segmental resection with stoma, Left portal ligature | Left hepatectomy extended to the right anterior sector (V, VIII) | — |
| **03** | Left colon | VI,VII,VIII | Left colectomy, Right portal ligation | Posterior sectectomy extended to VIII | — |
| **04** | Sigmoid | VI,VII,VIII | Low segmental resection, Right portal ligation | Right hepatectomy | — |
| **05** | Sigmoid | II,III,V,VIII | Low segmental resection, Wedge resection III, right portal ligation | Right hepatectomy , | — |

| | | | | metastasectomy II | |
|---|---|---|---|---|---|
| **06** | Sigmoid | III,V,VI,VII | Left colonic resection enlarged to the right with stoma + Deloyer, Metastasectomy III, right portal ligation | Right hepatectomy | — |

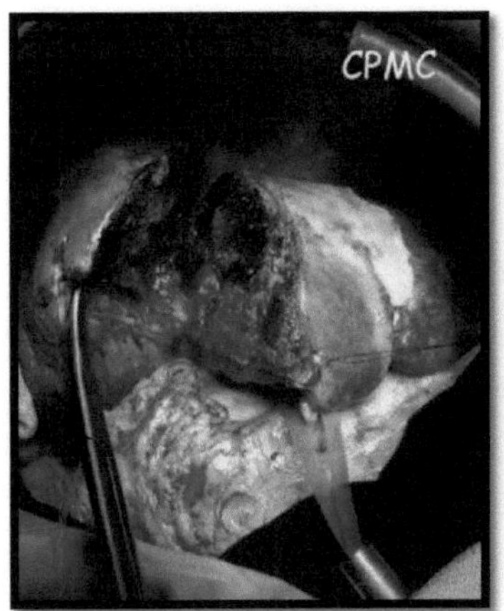

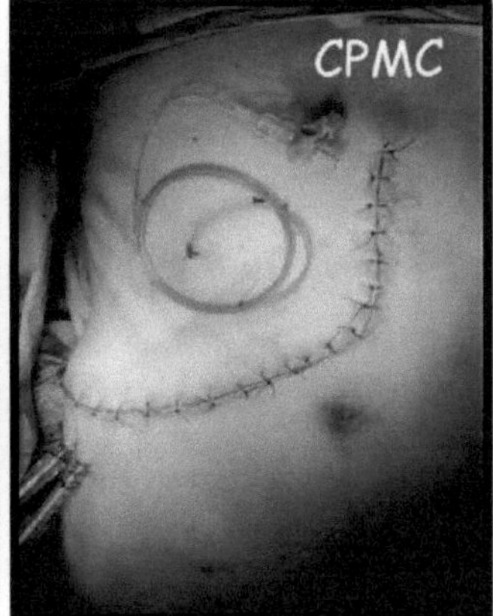


**Figure 41** First stage of ALPPS (CPMC).

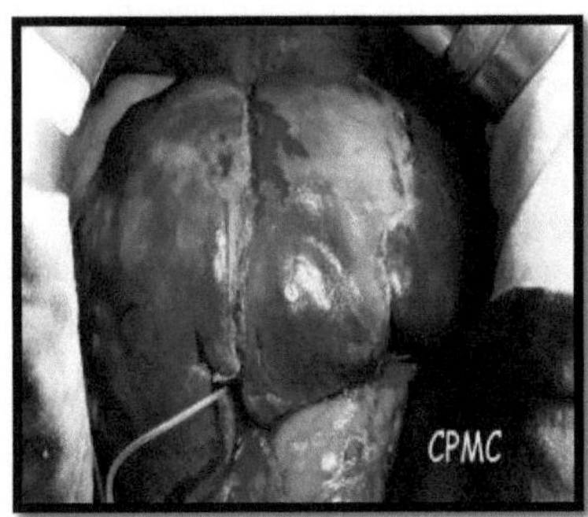

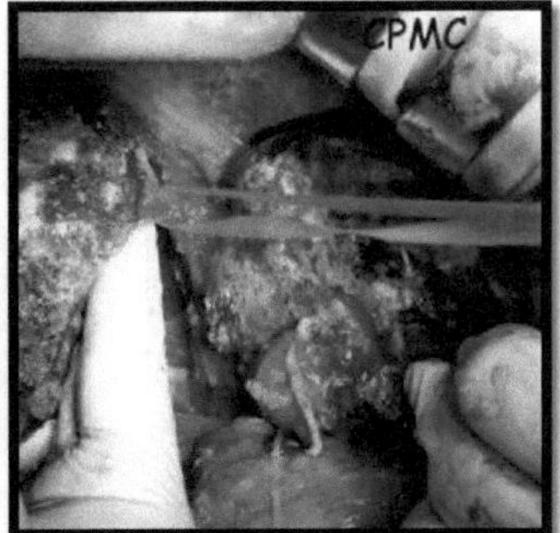


**Figure 42** Second stage of ALPPS (CPMC).

**Table 43** Volume gain after portal ligation and surgical interval.

| | Initial remaining liver volume | Liver volume remaining after portal ligation | Volume gain | Time between interventions | CT in the interval |
|---|---|---|---|---|---|
| **Patient 01** | 301.48 cc | 373.35cc / 507.38cc | 23,84 / 68,29% | 1ère -------2 ème 08 weeks 2ème ------3 ème 02 weeks | Yes |
| **Patient 02** | 304.52 cc | 509 cc | 67,14 % | 13 weeks | No |
| **Patient 03** | 312.2 cc | 313 cc | 0,26 % | 20 weeks | Yes |
| **Patient 04** | 394.58 cc | 517 cc | 31,02 % | 28 weeks | Yes |
| **Patient 05** | 383.34 cc | 622 cc | 62,25 % | 12 weeks | Yes |
| **Patient 06** | 382.84 cc | 645.90 cc | 68,71 % | 16 weeks | Yes |

After portal ligation, 5 of the 6 patients had significantly enlarged the remaining future liver, with a mean gain in volume of 59.48% (31.02% - 68.71%).
The absence of hepatic hypertrophy (0.26% gain in remaining liver volume) was noted in one patient. Despite this, the second hepatic stage was performed in this patient (posterior sectoriectomy enlarged to segment VIII) instead of a right hepatectomy, following a significant reduction in the volume of liver metastases under drug treatment.

In one patient, an additional hepatic partition was required after the portal ligation during a second operation, leading to a major hepatectomy (right hepatectomy) in a third operation (ALPPS) (Fig.41, Fig.42).
In the remaining patients, liver metastases were resected in two stages.

(Fig.43) and (Fig.44) show on a 3D reconstruction the hypertrophy of the future remaining liver in patient n°6.

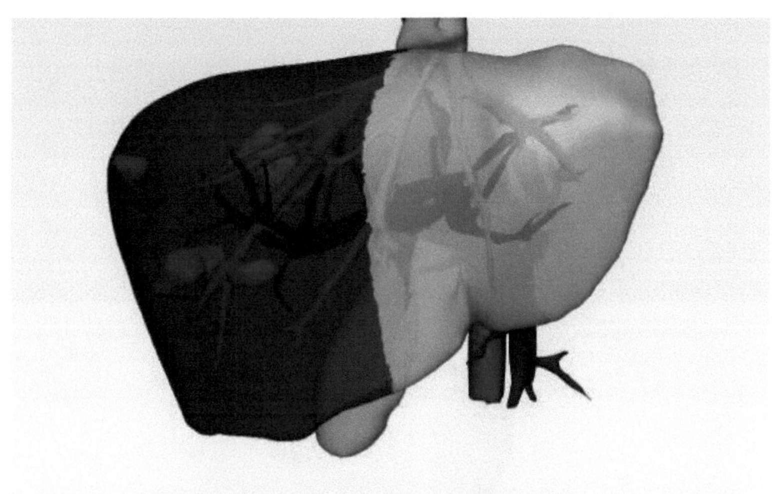

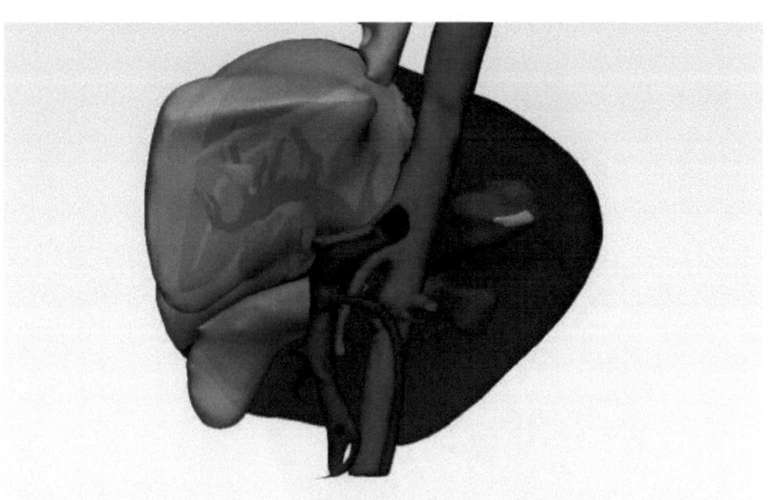

**Figure 43** 3D reconstruction with volumetry before portal ligation in Patient N°6 (note the single metastasis in the left lobe).

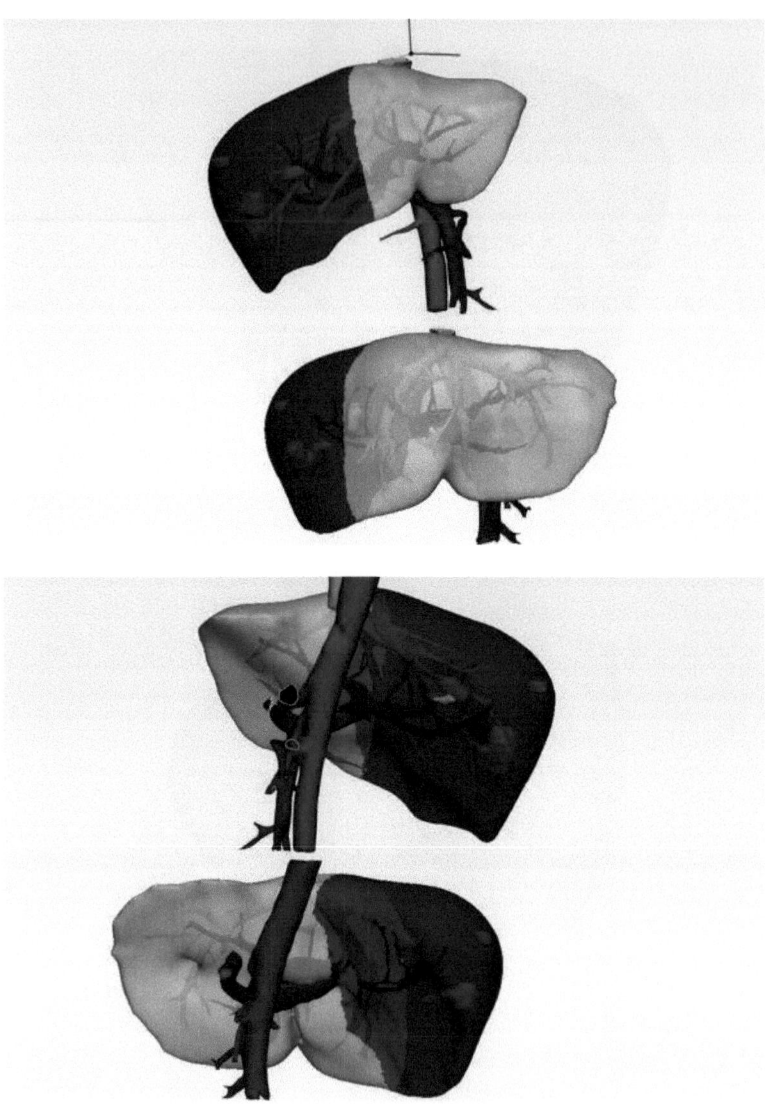

**Figure 44** Hypertrophy of the left liver after right portal ligation in patient n°6 (Note the metastasectomy scar (clearance of the left liver)).
(Anterior and posterior views showing the liver before and after Ligature).

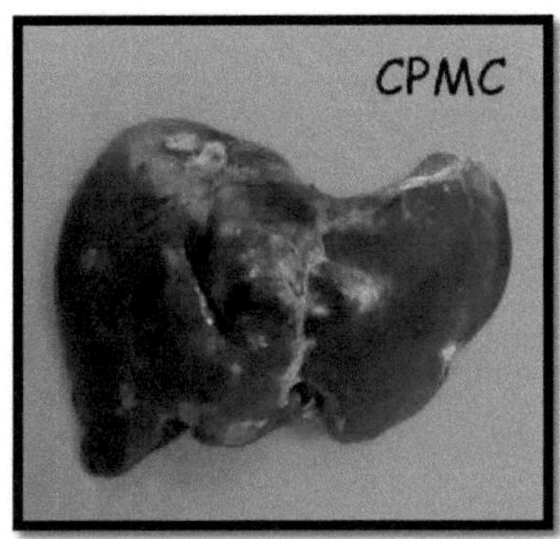

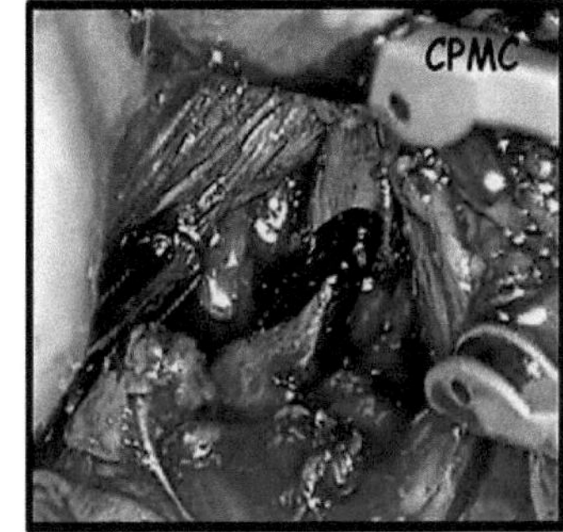


**Figure 45** Left hepatectomy extended to the right anterior sector after left portal ligation (patient no. 2) (CPMC).

Three patients had undergone a two-stage hepatectomy without prior portal ligation, and presented with bilobar liver metastases requiring multiple resections. During the first stage of surgery, a hybrid resection was performed, combining laparoscopic resection of the primary tumor with resection of part of the liver metastases, followed a few weeks later by surgery to remove the rest of the liver metastases by conventional means. In the interval between the two procedures, chemotherapy was administered.

**Table 44** Two-stage hepatectomies after hybrid surgery.

| | Primitive | Metastasis | First intervention | Second intervention | Time between procedures | CT in the interval |
|---|---|---|---|---|---|---|
| **07** | Sigmoid | III, IVa,VII,VIII | Low segment resection Wedge resection III | Wedge resection IVa, VII and VIII | 28 weeks | Yes |
| **08** | Upper rectum | II,III,IVb,V,VI,VII,VIII | RA+EPM+ACR Wedge resection III + Metastasectomy IV b+ Metastasectomy II-III | Sub-segmentectomy VI, sub-segmentectomy VII, metastasectomies V,VIII | 32 weeks | Yes |
| **09** | Sigmoid | II,IVa,IVb,V,VI,VII,VIII | Low segment resection Wedge resection II, IV b, metastasectomy VIII, wedge VI-VII | Wedge resection IVa, V Metastasectomy VI | 20 weeks | Yes |

6. **Morbidity:**

### *a) Intraoperative :*

### (1) Oslo classification :

Evaluated using the Oslo classification, which modified the Satava classification for intraoperative incidents (table 45).

**Table 45** Intraoperative incidents according to the Oslo classification.

| Grade | Number | Percentage |
|---|---|---|
| **1** | 04 | 10 % |
| **2** | 06 | 15 % |
| **3** | 00 | 00 % |
| **Total** | 10 | 25 % |

Intraoperative anesthetic or surgical incidents occurred in 10 patients, or 25% of the total. They were grade 1 in 4 patients and grade 2 in 6 patients.

Grade 1 incidents were as follows:
-Bladder wound at the insertion of the suprapubic trocar, requiring laparoscopic suture and bladder catheterization for 5 days.
-Rhythm disorders and extrasystoles at induction in ASA III cardiopaths (medically treated).
-Colonic perforation during extraction of the surgical specimen.
-Hypercapnia, which forced us to reduce insufflation pressures.

Grade 2 incidents were as follows:
-Impossible trocar placement due to adherent abdomen (conversion).
-Hypertensive peak with a mean arterial pressure (MAP) of 190mm hg which forced us to shorten the operative procedure.
-Hemodynamic problems due to poor tolerance of pneumoperitoneum, which forced us to convert.
-Injury to Riolan's arch during an anterior resection, which forced us to extend the colonic resection procedure.
-Colonic wound that had been sutured and then washed away in the resection.
-Hemorrhagic incident requiring transfusion.

Statistical analysis of possible factors influencing the occurrence of an intraoperative incident is summarized in Table 46, and of a severe Oslo 2 incident in Table 47.

**Table 46** Risk factors for the occurrence of an intraoperative incident.

| | *p* value |
|---|---|
| **Age** | 0,270 |
| **Gender** | 0,293 |
| **Comorbidities (ASA II, III)** | **0,049** |
| **Previous abdominal surgery** | 0,165 |
| **Previous median incision** | 0,089 |
| **BMI** | 0,433 |
| **Primitive (colon/rectum)** | 0,132 |
| **Operating time** | 0,719 |

**Table 47** Risk factors for the occurrence of a severe intraoperative incident.

| | *p* value |
|---|---|
| **Age** | 0,649 |
| **Gender** | 0,676 |
| **Comorbidities (ASA II ,III)** | 0,174 |
| **Previous abdominal surgery** | **0,037** |
| **Previous median incision** | **0,013** |
| **BMI** | 0,174 |
| **Primitive (colon/rectum)** | 0,646 |
| **Operating time** | 0,101 |

The occurrence of an intraoperative incident was statistically linked to the presence of comorbidities ($p = 0.049$).

The occurrence of a severe incident (Oslo 2) was related to previous abdominal surgery, especially if the anterior incision was a midline incision ($p = 0.013$).

### (2) Intraoperative transfusion :

Three patients had been transfused intraoperatively, including one after a bleeding incident (mentioned above).
The characteristics of transfused patients (age and terrain), surgery and preoperative hemoglobin levels are summarized in Table 48.

**Table 48** Patients transfused intraoperatively.

| | Age | Land | Intervention | Type | Incident | Conversion | Duration | Preoperative Hb level | Output |
|---|---|---|---|---|---|---|---|---|---|
| 01 | 63 | ASA I | RA+ETM+ACSA+ileostomy+right annexectomy, metastasectomy III | All laparoscopic | + | - | 310 mn | 8.2 g/dl | J04 |
| 02 | 66 | ASA II Diabetes, cardiopathy | Low segmental resection, Double metastasectomy IVa, VIII | Hybrid surgery | - | - | 270 mn | 9.9 g/dl | J05 |
| 03 | 65 | ASA II HTA | RA+ETM+ACA+ ileostomy, Wedge straddle resection VI,VII | Hybrid surgery | + | - | 360 minutes | 13.7 g/dl | J04 |

The transfusion volume was two packed red blood cells for patients 01 and 02 at the end of the procedure.
For patient 03, the transfusion volume was a single packed red blood cell during the procedure (hemorrhagic incident).
No transfusion-related complications were noted.

### *b) Postoperative morbidity:*

#### (1) Thirty days :

Thirty-day morbidity expressed according to the Clavien-Dindo-Strasberg classification is summarized in Table 49, with details of postoperative complications presented according to the "Japan Clinical Oncology Group postoperative complications criteria" gradation.

**Table 49** 30-day morbidity according to the Clavien-Dindo-Strasberg classification.

| Post-operative complications | Clavien-Dindo-Strasberg classification | | | | | |
|---|---|---|---|---|---|---|
| | Grade I | Grade II | Grade III a | Grade III b | Grade IV a | Grade IV b |
| Pneumopathy | | 1 | | | | |

| Vomiting | 1 | | | | | |
|---|---|---|---|---|---|---|
| Transfusion | | 1 | | | | |
| Wall sepsis | | 1 | | | | |
| Collection | | | 1 | 1 | | |
| Gastroparesis | | 1 | | | | |
| Grade B fistula | | 1 | | | | |
| Dehydration | 1 | | | | | |
| Urinary catheter (wound) | 1 | | | | | |
| Tachyarrhythmia | 1 | | | | | |
| Total = 11 | 4 | 5 | 1 | 1 | 0 | 0 |
| 11/40 (27,5%) | 09/40 (22,5%) | | 2/40 (5%) | | | |
| 11 (100%) | 09/11 (81,82 %) | | 2/11 (18,18 %) | | | |

Overall morbidity at 30 days was 27.5%, represented mainly by mild morbidity (Clavien Grade I and II).

This mild morbidity affected 09 patients, representing 22.5% of the total study population, and 81.82% of patients with morbidity.

For grade I morbidity (4 patients) we noted :

-A patient who had experienced prolonged postoperative vomiting, necessitating prescription of antiemetics and adequate rehydration, with a prolonged postoperative stay (discharge at D 07).

-A diabetic, hypertensive patient with an ileostomy who had been readmitted at D 26 postoperatively for dehydration. A 48-hour hospital stay was required to correct the disorders.

-A patient whose bladder catheterization with a Foley catheter had been held for five days following a bladder wound at the insertion of the suprapubic trocar, which had required laparoscopic suturing.

A diabetic patient with post-surgical hypoparathyroidism presented with postoperative tachycardia associated with arrhythmia, requiring intensive care monitoring and treatment.

**Table 50** Grade I morbidity.

| | Age | Land | Intervention | Type | Incident | Conversion | Duration | Morbidity | Output |
|---|---|---|---|---|---|---|---|---|---|
| 01 | 32 | ASA I | RA+EPM+ACR, wedge resection VII | Hybrid Surgery | - | - | 290 min. | Vomiting | J 07 |
| 02 | 72 | ASA II | RA+ETM+ACSA +iléostomie, Sub-segmentectomy VI, Metastasectomy VII | Hybrid Surgery | - | - | 420 mn | Dehydration | J05 Readmission J02 |
| 03 | 64 | ASA II | RA+EPM+ACR+ wedge resection III | All laparoscopic | + | - | 300 mn | Bladder probe | J 05 |
| 04 | 72 | ASA II Diabetes | right hemicolectomy, wedge resection straddling segments V and VI | Laparotomy | + | + | 240 minutes | Tachyarrhythmia | J 06 |

For grade II morbidity (5 patients) we noted :

-A diabetic patient who presented with a pulmonary infection (left basal lung disease) requiring antibiotic treatment (discharged at D 05).

-A patient who presented with wall sepsis on a Makuuchi incision associated with cellulitis of the right flank that required local care plus initiation of antibiotic therapy (Discharged at D13).

-A patient who presented with a grade B anastomotic fistula (appendix 7) on a protected colo-sus-anal anastomosis, discovered on imaging (CT scan with digestive opacification) requested at D15 following a painful symptomatology, treated medically on an outpatient basis with a favorable outcome.

-A patient who had required a postoperative transfusion of two packed red blood cells, following bleeding externalized by drainage with a fall in hemoglobin to 6.8 g/dl.

-A patient who had presented with gastroparesis requiring placement of a nasogastric tube (discharged at D07).

**Table 51** Grade II morbidity.

| | Age | Land | Intervention | Type | Incident | Conversion | Duration | Morbidity | Output |
|---|---|---|---|---|---|---|---|---|---|
| 01 | 58 | ASA II Diabetes, hypertension | Left colonic resection, wedge resection III | Hybrid Surgery | - | - | 355 mn | Pneumopathy | J 05 |
| 02 | 61 | ASA I | Right hemicolectomy, Sub-segmentectomy VII, double | Hybrid Surgery | - | - | 360 minutes | Wall sepsis + cellulitis | J13 |

| | | | | | | | | | |
|---|---|---|---|---|---|---|---|---|---|
| | | | metastasectomy VII, scar resection VI | | | | | | |
| 03 | 58 | ASA I | RA+ETM+ACSA +ileostomy, metastasectomy III, IVa | All laparoscopic | - | - | 360 minutes | Grade B fistula | J04 |
| 04 | 35 | ASA I | Low segmental resection, Wedge resection II, IV b, metastasectomy VIII, wedge VI-VII | Downstaging surgery | - | - | 370 mn | Post-operative transfusion | J07 |
| 05 | 65 | ASA I | Enlarged total colectomy, double metastasectomy VII VIII | Laparotomy | - | + | 270 mn | Gastroparesis | J07 |

Severe morbidity affected 02 patients, representing 5% of the total study population, and 15.38% of patients with morbidity.

For grade IIIa morbidity we noted :
-A patient who had been readmitted at D11 postoperatively for a collection in the hepatectomy pocket, diagnosed on CT scan as part of the etiological exploration of an infectious syndrome, (9×10×8 cm hydroaeric collection), this collection had been drained radiologically under local anaesthesia, and antibiotic therapy had been instituted. Radiological control at [48] hours was satisfactory. The evolution was favorable (discharge at J02).

For grade IIIb morbidity we noted :
-A diabetic hypertensive patient presented with a deep abdominal collection diagnosed on CT scan as part of the etiological exploration of an infectious syndrome. Surgical abdominal revision was performed at D11 postoperatively, and drainage of the collection and peritoneal cleansing were performed. The evolution was favorable (discharge at D17).

**Table 52** Grade III morbidity.

| | Age | Land | Intervention | Type | Incident | Conversion | Duration | Morbidity | Output |
|---|---|---|---|---|---|---|---|---|---|
| 01 | 63 | ASA II | Right hemicolectomy, segmentectomy VII | Hybrid Surgery | - | - | 300 mn | Hepatectomy loge collection. Radiological drainage at D11 | J 05 Readmission J02 |

| 02 | 61 | ASA II Diabetes, hypertension | Left colorectal resection enlarged to the right + Deloyer, Wedge straddle resection VI,VII | Hybrid Surgery | + | - | 360 minutes | Intra-abdominal collection. Surgical revision at D11 | J17 |
|---|---|---|---|---|---|---|---|---|---|

During the one-month post-operative period, two readmissions (described above) were noted, corresponding to a readmission rate of 5%.

### (2) At ninety days :

In the ninety postoperative days, an additional morbidity was noted, and had concerned a 70-year-old patient, ASA II (HTA) operated on for adenocarcinoma of the middle rectum with single hepatic metastasis of segment IVb. An anterior resection (with total removal of the mesorectum and latero-terminal mechanical colo-sus-anal anastomosis protected by an ileostomy) had been performed, combined with an IVb segmentectomy. The early postoperative course was favourable, and the patient was discharged on postoperative day 04.
A systematic follow-up TAP CT scan performed at D38 postoperatively revealed a 32×61×60 mm presacral collection in contact with the posterior surface of the anastomosis, associated with an 84×76×95 mm hydroaeric collection of the hepatic resection pocket.
We considered that the patient had presented with a grade A anastomotic fistula since he was asymptomatic, and we delayed closure of the ileostomy for three months.
The collection in the hepatectomy pocket had been drained radiologically on an outpatient basis, and the bacteriological study of the fluid sampled was negative.

### *c) Morbidity related to the second hepatic stage :*

Nine patients had undergone a second hepatic stage, including six after portal ligation. A major hepatic resection was performed in these six patients. The other three underwent multiple liver resections.
Morbidity related to major hepatectomy procedures was noted and involved three patients:
-A patient who presented with a postoperative collection of the hepatectomy lodge after the second stage of ALPPS, which necessitated repeat surgery (toilet plus drainage) with a favorable outcome.
-A patient who presented with an anastomotic fistula after left hepatectomy enlarged to the right anterior sector and bilio-biliary anastomosis.
This fistula had caused postoperative peritonitis, necessitating revision surgery. It developed into an external biliary fistula, which dried up after a few weeks.
-A cardiopathic patient (coronary stented in 2014, hypertensive) who had required a blood transfusion postoperatively after a right hepatectomy. Preoperative hemoglobin level was 12.5 g/dl. On D0 of the operation, the hemoglobin level was 10.5 g/dl and had dropped to 8.3 g/dl on D 02 postoperatively, necessitating a transfusion of two packed red blood cells.

## 7. Length of hospital stay :

Postoperative hospital stay averaged 5.1 ± 2.58 days with a median of 4 days and extremes of 3 and 17 days.

Depending on the type of surgical procedure, the length of hospital stay is summarized in (table 53) :

**Table 53** Length of postoperative stay by type of surgery.

| Type of surgery | Length of hospital stay in days | Number | *p* value |
|---|---|---|---|
| **All laparoscopic** | 4,25 ± 0,5 | 04 | 0,819 |
| **Hybrid Surgery** | 5,45 ± 3,17 | 24 | 0,206 |
| **Down staging surgery** | 4,33 ± 1,11 | 09 | 0,554 |
| **Conversion** | 5,66 ± 1,52 | 03 | 0,416 |
| **Total** | 5,1 ±2,58 | 40 | |

Eight patients underwent post-operative care in the intensive care unit, with an average stay of 3.75 days and a median of 2.5 days, with extremes ranging from 1 to 13 days.

## 8. Postoperative mortality:

Postoperative mortality at 30 days was nil.

## 9. Pathological anatomy :

The results of pathological analysis of the surgical specimens (colorectal resection, liver resection) were as follows:

### *a) Tumor size :*

**Table 54** Tumour size in millimetres.

| | Average tumor size |
|---|---|
| **Primary tumor** | 38 mm (10 to 90 mm) |
| **Liver metastasis** | 17.02 mm (2 to 55 mm) |

### *b) Histological type :*

**Table 55** Histological type of primary colorectal tumour.

| Histological type | Number | percentage |
|---|---|---|
| **Adenocarcinoma** | 36 | 90 % |
| **Mucinous adenocarcinoma** | 03 | 7,5 % |

| Full answer | 01 | 2,5 % |
|---|---|---|
| Total | 40 | 100 % |

**Table 56** Histological type of liver metastasis.

| Histological type | Number | percentage |
|---|---|---|
| Adenocarcinoma | 28 | 80 % |
| Mucinous adenocarcinoma | 01 | 2,86 % |
| Full answer | 06 | 17,14 % |
| Total | 35 | 100 % |

### *c) Differentiation :*

**Table 57** Degree of differentiation of the primary tumor.

| Differentiation | Number | percentage |
|---|---|---|
| Fine | 20 | 50 % |
| Medium | 16 | 40 % |
| Little | 00 | 00 % |
| Mucinous | 03 | 7,5 % |
| Full answer | 01 | 2,5 % |
| Total | 40 | 100 % |

**Table 58** Degree of differentiation of liver metastasis.

| Differentiation | Number | percentage |
|---|---|---|
| Fine | 10 | 28,57 % |
| Medium | 04 | 11,43 % |
| Little | 00 | 00 % |
| Mucinous | 01 | 2,86 % |
| Full answer | 06 | 17,14 % |
| Not specified | 14 | 40 % |
| Total | 35 | 100 % |

### *d) Resection margins :*

Resection margins were calculated on 40 colorectal resection specimens and 56 liver resection specimens.

**Table 59** Surgical resection margins.

| Resection margins | Healthy | <1mm |
|---|---|---|
| Primary tumor : | | |
| Proximal | 40 | 00 |

| Distal | 40 | 00 |
|---|---|---|
| Circumferential | 38 | 02 |
| Liver metastasis | 52 | 04 |

### e) *Mesorectal quality :*

The mesorectum was complete Quirke grade 3 on all 16 rectal resections performed.

### f) *Number of nodes in curage :*

The mean number of nodes in the curage was 15.55, with a median of 12.5 and extremes ranging from 1 to 54 nodes.

**Table 60** Average number of nodes in curage.

| | Average number of nodes(gg) | | *p* value |
|---|---|---|---|
| The whole series (40) | 15.55 gg | | |
| Neoadjuvant treatments | Yes (34) | No (06) | |
| | 14.56 gg | 21.17 gg | 0,176 |
| Preoperative chemotherapy | Yes (29) | No (11) | |
| | 13.31 gg | 21.45 gg | **0,034** |

The mean number of lymph nodes in the curage was compared between patients who had received neoadjuvant treatment (34 patients) and those who had undergone immediate surgery (06 patients) (table 60).
The mean number of nodes in the curage was compared between patients who had received preoperative chemotherapy (29 patients) and patients operated on without prior chemotherapy (11 patients) (table 60).

The number of nodes in the curage was significantly lower in the case of preoperative chemotherapy.

### g) *Therapeutic response:*

Therapeutic response to neoadjuvant treatment was assessed for the primary tumor according to the RCRG classification, and for liver metastasis according to the TRG classification.

**Table 61** Therapeutic response of primary tumor according to RCRG.

| Therapeutic response | RCRG 1 | RCRG2 | RCRG3 | NP | Total |
|---|---|---|---|---|---|
| Primary tumor | 02 | 10 | 13 | 09 | 34 |

**Table 62** Therapeutic response of liver metastasis according to TRG.

| Therapeutic response | TRG 1 | TRG2 | TRG3 | TRG4 | TRG5 | NP | Total |
|---|---|---|---|---|---|---|---|
| **Liver metastasis** | 06 | 06 | 06 | 03 | 00 | 08 | 29 |

### *h) pTNM classification :*

**Table 63** pTNM classification.

| Classification | Number |
|---|---|
| T0N0M1 | 01 (2,5 %) |
| T1N0M1a | 01 (2,5 %) |
| T2N0M1a | 01 (2,5 %) |
| **T3N0M1a** | **16 (40 %)** |
| **T3$N_{1-2}$M1a** | **20 (50 %)** |
| T4$N_{1-2}$M1a | 01 (2,5 %) |
| Total | 40 (100 %) |

### *i) UICC stadiums :*

All patients were classified as UICC stage IVA.

## 10. **Follow-up:**

Patient follow-up averaged 15 months, with a median of 12.5 months and extremes ranging from 2 months to 41 months.
Follow-up was carried out in consultation, and the events noted were essentially the occurrence of a recurrence of the cancerous disease or a distant complication.

### a) *Recurrences :*

Nine patients (22.5% of the total) had experienced a recurrence of their cancer after curative treatment.
The type as well as the time to recurrence and our conduct are summarized in Table 64 :

**Table 64** Recurrences (type, delay and treatment).

| Patient | Type of recurrence | Delay | CAT | Survival |
|---|---|---|---|---|
| Colon + MH Hybrid | Single epiploic nodule positive on PET scan | 13 months | Laparoscopic resection + CT | Alive at 37 months |
| Colon + MH (ALLPS) | Single liver metastasis | 14 months | rehepatectomy | Alive at 25 months |
| Rectum + MH Hybrid | MH + Bilateral lung metastases | 17 months | CT | Alive at 21 months |
| Colon + MH Hybrid | MH + Ganglion | 10 months | CT | Alive at 19 months |
| Colon + MH Down staging | MH | 27 months | CT | Alive at 30 months |
| Colon + MH Down staging | MH | 22 months | CT | Alive at 26 months |
| Rectum + MH All coelio | MH | 06 months | CT | Alive at 12 months |
| Colon + MH Hybrid | Bone metastasis | 09 months | CT | Alive at 12 months |
| Rectum +MH Hybrid | MH | 04 months | CT (awaiting resection) | Alive at 4 months |

**Table 65** Characteristics of patients with recurrence.

| | Location | Intervention | Morbidity | PTNM | Residue |
|---|---|---|---|---|---|
| **01** | Left colon + segment III | Left colectomy + wedge resection III (hybrid) | Grade I | pT3N1aM1a | R0 |

| **02** | Sigmoid+ segments II,III,VI,VII,VIII | Down staging then ALPPS | - | ypT3N2aM1a | R0 |
|---|---|---|---|---|---|
| **03** | Rectum + segment IVb | RA + segmentectomy IVb | Grade IIIa | ypT3N1aM1a | R0 |
| **04** | Sigmoid + segments IVb,VI | Low segmental resection + segmentectomy IVb, wedge VI | - | ypT3N1aM1a | R0 |
| **05** | Sigmoid + segments III, IVa,VII,VIII | Low segment resection + wedge III 2ème multiple resections | - | ypT3N1aM1a | R1 Liver (2ème time) |
| **06** | Sigmoid + segments II,IV,V,VIII | Low segmental resection + left portal ligation 2ème left hepatectomy + anterior sector | - | ypT3N0M1a | R1 Liver (2ème time) |
| **07** | Upper rectum + segment III | RA + wedge III All coelio | - | pT3N2aM1a | R1 Rectum |
| **08** | Left colon + segments VI,VII | Low segmental resection + straddle wedge VI, VII | - | ypT1N0M1a | R0 |
| **09** | Lower rectum + segment IVb | PAA + IVb segmentectomy | - | ypT3N2bM1a | R0 |

### *b) Remote complications :*

Two of our patients had a remote complication in the form of eventration:
- One patient presented with a peristomal eventration after PAA.
- One patient presented with a median eventration on Makuuchi incision.

### *c) Deaths :*

Postoperative mortality was nil.
No remote deaths were recorded.
All patients (N=40) were alive at the point date 26/01/2020.

## 11. Survival study :

a) ***Overall survival***: All patients were alive at baseline. Median follow-up was 12.5 months, with extremes ranging from 02 to 41 months.

### *b) Recurrence-free survival :*

During the surveillance period, nine patients had relapsed.
Mean recurrence-free survival was 28.91 months.
Median recurrence-free survival was 27 months.

**Table 66** Means and medians for recurrence-free survival.

| Average | | | | Median | | | |
|---|---|---|---|---|---|---|---|
| Estimate | Standard error | 95% confidence interval | | Estimate | Standard error | 95% confidence interval | |
| | | Lower terminal | Upper terminal | | | Lower terminal | Upper terminal |
| 28,918 | 3,125 | 22,792 | 35,044 | 27,000 | . | . | . |

The recurrence-free survival curve is as follows:

### (1) Recurrence-free survival curve for the series:

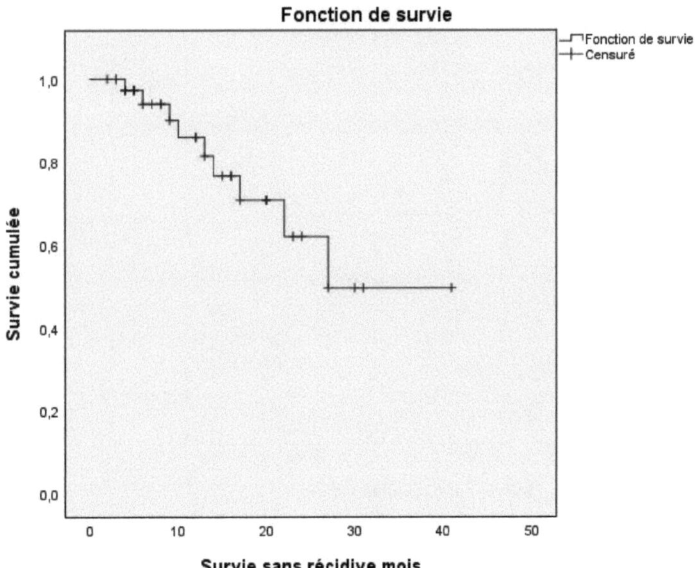


**Figure 46** Recurrence-free survival curve for the series.

### (2) Recurrence-free survival curve by gender :

Mean recurrence-free survival was 26.22 months in men and 24.88 months in women, with no significant difference $p = 0.605$.

**Table 67** Means and medians for recurrence-free survival by gender.

| Sex 1F/0H | Average | | | | Median | | | |
|---|---|---|---|---|---|---|---|---|
| | Estimate | Standard error | 95% confidence interval | | Estimate | Standard error | 95% confidence interval | |
| | | | Lower terminal | Upper terminal | | | Lower terminal | Upper terminal |
| 0 | 26,223 | 3,978 | 18,426 | 34,021 | 27,000 | 5,409 | 16,399 | 37,601 |
| 1 | 24,889 | 3,037 | 18,936 | 30,842 | . | . | . | . |
| Global | 28,918 | 3,125 | 22,792 | 35,044 | 27,000 | . | . | . |

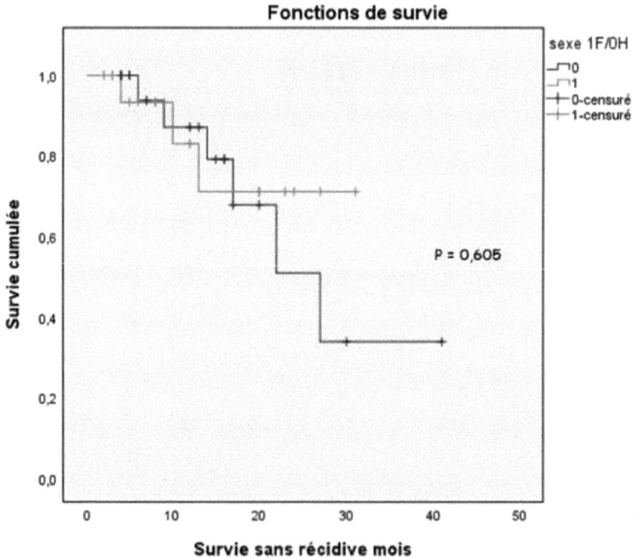


**Figure 47** Recurrence-free survival curve by gender.

### (3) Recurrence-free survival curve by age :

Mean recurrence-free survival was 28.88 months for age ≤ 65 years and 20.75 months for age > 65 years, with no significant difference *p* = 0.787.

**Table 68** Means and medians for recurrence-free survival by age.

| Age range ≤ 65 (0), > 65 (1) | Average | | | | Median | | | |
|---|---|---|---|---|---|---|---|---|
| | Estimate | Standard error | 95% confidence interval | | Estimate | Standard error | 95% confidence interval | |
| | | | Lower terminal | Upper terminal | | | Lower terminal | Upper terminal |
| 0 | 28,885 | 3,596 | 21,837 | 35,933 | . | . | . | . |
| 1 | 20,750 | 1,531 | 17,749 | 23,751 | 22,000 | ,000 | . | . |
| Global | 28,918 | 3,125 | 22,792 | 35,044 | 27,000 | . | . | . |

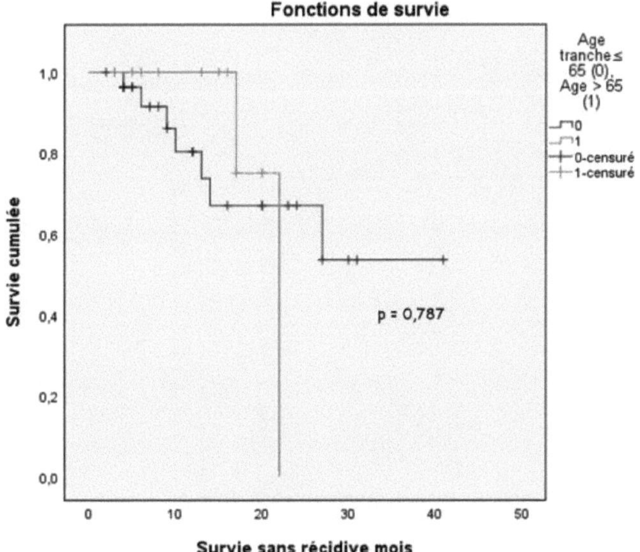


**Figure 48** Recurrence-free survival curve by age .

## (4) Recurrence-free survival curve according to CEA level :

Mean recurrence-free survival was 26.9 months for normal CEA levels and 26.57 months for high CEA levels, with no significant difference $p = 0.334$.

**Table 69** Means and medians for recurrence-free survival according to CEA level.

| ACE standards 0, high 1 | Average | | | | Median | | | |
|---|---|---|---|---|---|---|---|---|
| | Estimate | Standard error | 95% confidence interval | | Estimate | Standard error | 95% confidence interval | |
| | | | Lower terminal | Upper terminal | | | Lower terminal | Upper terminal |
| 0 | 26,905 | 2,607 | 21,796 | 32,014 | . | . | . | . |
| 1 | 26,577 | 3,810 | 19,110 | 34,044 | 27,000 | 8,516 | 10,308 | 43,692 |
| Global | 28,918 | 3,125 | 22,792 | 35,044 | 27,000 | . | . | . |

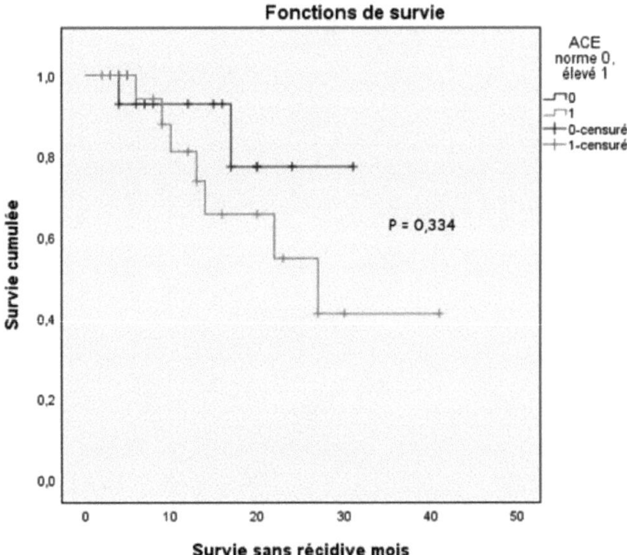


**Figure 49** Recurrence-free survival curve according to CEA level.

### (5) Recurrence-free survival curve by primary tumor location :

Mean recurrence-free survival was 27.63 months for colonic primitives and 23.82 months for rectal primitives, with no significant difference $p = 0.923$.

**Table 70** Means and medians for recurrence-free survival by primary tumor location.

| Primary tumor colon 0, rectum 1 | Average | | | | Median | | | |
|---|---|---|---|---|---|---|---|---|
| | Estimate | Standard error | 95% confidence interval | | Estimate | Standard error | 95% confidence interval | |
| | | | Lower terminal | Upper terminal | | | Lower terminal | Upper terminal |
| 0 | 27,632 | 3,851 | 20,083 | 35,180 | 27,000 | 4,917 | 17,363 | 36,637 |
| 1 | 23,825 | 3,488 | 16,989 | 30,661 | . | . | . | . |
| Global | 28,918 | 3,125 | 22,792 | 35,044 | 27,000 | . | . | . |

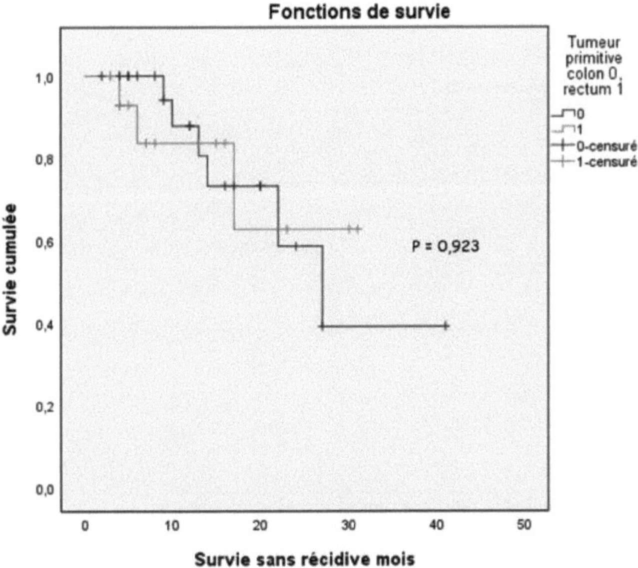


**Figure 50** Recurrence-free survival curve by primary tumor location.

## (6) Recurrence-free survival curve according to lymph node infiltration :

Mean recurrence-free survival was 34.15 months in the absence of lymph node infiltration and 20.92 months in the presence of lymph node infiltration, with no significant difference $p = 0.088$.

**Table 71** Mean and median recurrence-free survival according to lymph node infiltration.

| pN N0 (0) N+(1) | Average | | | | Median | | | |
|---|---|---|---|---|---|---|---|---|
| | Estimate | Standard error | 95% confidence interval | | Estimate | Standard error | 95% confidence interval | |
| | | | Lower terminal | Upper terminal | | | Lower terminal | Upper terminal |
| 0 | 34,154 | 4,298 | 25,729 | 42,578 | . | . | . | . |
| 1 | 20,927 | 2,753 | 15,531 | 26,323 | 27,000 | 8,088 | 11,147 | 42,853 |
| Global | 28,918 | 3,125 | 22,792 | 35,044 | 27,000 | . | . | . |

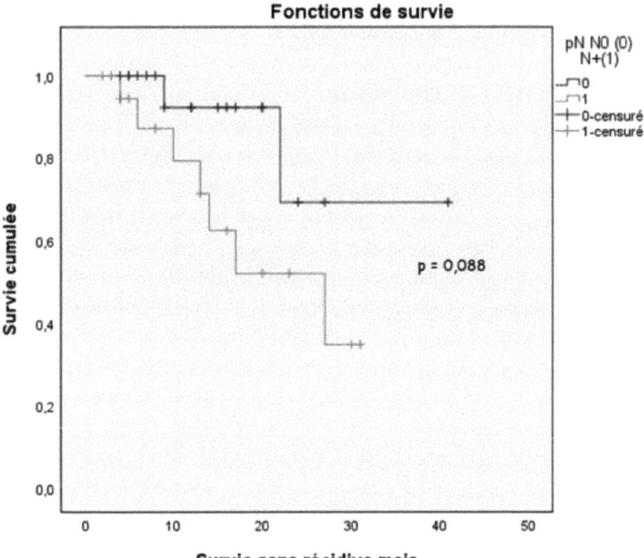


**Figure 51** Recurrence-free survival curve according to lymph node infiltration.

### (7) Recurrence-free survival curve according to whether surgery was R0 or R1 :

Mean recurrence-free survival was 28.71 months with R0 surgery and 18.75 months with R1 surgery, with no significant difference $p = 0.964$.

**Table 72** Means and medians for recurrence-free survival according to whether surgery was R0 or R1.

| R0(0) R1(1) | Average | | | | Median | | | |
|---|---|---|---|---|---|---|---|---|
| | Estimate | Standard error | 95% confidence interval | | Estimate | Standard error | 95% confidence interval | |
| | | | Lower terminal | Upper terminal | | | Lower terminal | Upper terminal |
| 0 | 28,717 | 3,278 | 22,292 | 35,141 | 27,000 | . | . | . |
| 1 | 18,750 | 3,681 | 11,536 | 25,964 | . | . | . | . |
| Global | 28,918 | 3,125 | 22,792 | 35,044 | 27,000 | . | . | . |

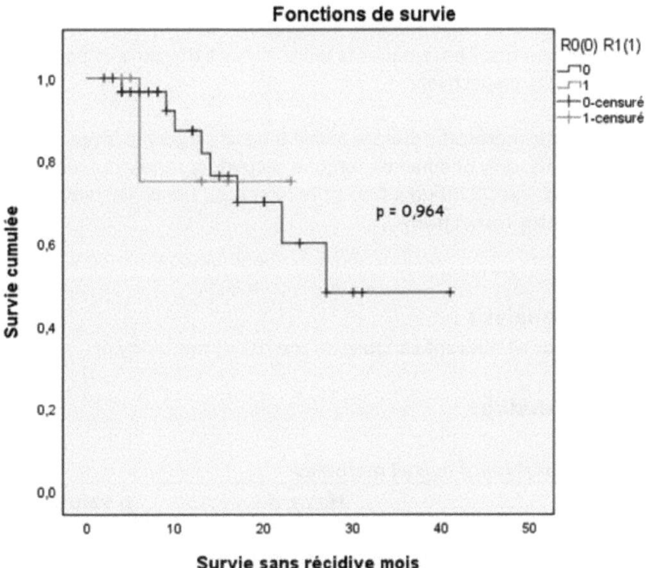


**Figure 52** Recurrence-free survival curve according to R0 or R1.

## 12. **Outcome of excluded patients :**

Ten patients who met the inclusion criteria were excluded secondarily.

Four patients did not undergo surgery and were excluded from the study due to progression of their metastatic disease on chemotherapy.
They had continued with drug treatment (chemotherapy + targeted therapy).
Two died at 03 months and 12 months respectively from the start of treatment.

Two were alive at baseline, at 07 months and 09 months respectively from the start of treatment.

Six other patients had undergone laparoscopic surgery but were excluded from the study for various reasons (Fig.30) :

- One patient was found to have generalized peritoneal carcinosis during laparoscopic exploration. He continued his drug treatment until his death 12 months postoperatively.

- Laparoscopic surgery to remove the primary tumor without approaching the liver in five patients for :

-Diagnostic error: cystic or angiomatous liver lesions initially labelled as liver metastases in two patients. These patients were alive at the time of point at 06 months and 09 months respectively.

-Progression of hepatic metastatic disease at the time of surgery in three patients. Of these three patients, only one had undergone secondary surgery to remove his liver metastases, and was 12 months free of recurrence. The other two patients died at 8 and 16 months respectively.

## 13. Univariate analysis :

We studied the role of all relevant variables in the risk of morbidity or recurrence.

### *a) Overall morbidity :*

**Table 73** Univariate analysis of overall morbidity.

| Variable | Hazard ratio | *p* value |
|---|---|---|
| **Gender** | 1,964 | 0,276 |
| **Age (≤65 />65)** | 0,494 | 0,349 |
| **BMI (<25/≥25)** | 0,703 | 0,454 |
| **ASA comorbidities** | **3,325** | 0,096 |
| **Anemia symptom** | **7,714** | **0,039** |
| **Previous abdominal surgery** | 1,270 | 0,514 |
| **Primitive (colon/rectum)** | 1,364 | 0,467 |
| **Metastasis (single/multiple)** | 0,847 | 0,586 |
| **Unilobar/bilobar** | 0,190 | 0,110 |
| **Metastasis size** | - | 0,660 |
| **All laparoscopic** | 3,000 | 0,300 |
| **Hybrid surgery** | 0,733 | 0,467 |

| | | |
|---|---|---|
| **Down staging surgery** | 0,263 | 0,209 |
| **Neoadjuvant treatment** | 0,130 | **0,039** |
| **Preoperative chemo** | 0,174 | **0,027** |
| **Number of chemotherapy treatments** | - | 0,166 |
| **Neoadjuvant radiotherapy** | 0,583 | 0,432 |
| **Hemoglobin < 10 g/dl** | 1,926 | 0,422 |
| **Albumin level (<35/≥35)** | 0,314 | 0,279 |
| **Tumor differentiation on biopsy** | - | 0,232 |
| **cT (TNM)** | 0,741 | 0,630 |
| **cN+ (TNM)** | - | 0,180 |
| **Portal ligature** | - | 0,124 |
| **Type of resection** | | |
| **Primary tumor** | - | 0,137 |
| **Metastasis** | - | 0,284 |
| **Number of resections** | - | **0,035** |
| **Clamping** | 0,422 | 0,275 |
| **Duration op** | - | 0,381 |
| **Incidents (Oslo)** | - | **0,045** |
| **Intraoperative transfusion** | - | 0,310 |
| **Conversion** | **6,222** | 0,178 |
| **Post-operative stay** | - | **0,030** |

***b) Mild morbidity: Clavien I, II :***

**Table 74** Univariate analysis for mild morbidity.

| Variable | Hazard ratio | *p* |
|---|---|---|
| **Gender** | 1,979 | 0,301 |
| **Age (≤65 />65)** | 0,698 | 0,523 |
| **BMI (<25/≥25)** | 0,607 | 0,406 |
| **ASA comorbidities** | 1,979 | 0,301 |
| **Anemia symptom** | **11,600** | **0,016** |
| **Previous abdominal surgery** | 1,050 | 0,624 |
| **Primitive (colon/rectum)** | 1,267 | 0,525 |
| **Metastasis (single/multiple)** | 0,903 | 0,594 |
| **Unilobar/bilobar** | 0,263 | 0,209 |
| **metastasis size** | - | 0,595 |
| **All laparoscopic** | 4,143 | 0,213 |

| | | |
|---|---|---|
| **Hybrid Surgery** | 0,440 | 0,242 |
| **Down staging surgery** | 0,359 | 0,333 |
| **Neoadjuvant treatment** | 0,086 | **0,016** |
| **Preoperative chemotherapy** | 0,096 | **0,007** |
| **Number of chemotherapy treatments** | - | 0,174 |
| **Neoadjuvant radiotherapy** | 0,821 | 0,601 |
| **Hemoglobin < 10 g/dl** | 2,667 | 0,311 |
| **Albumin level (<35/≥35)** | 0,429 | 0,410 |
| **Tumor differentiation on biopsy** | - | 0,171 |
| **cT (TNM)** | 0,552 | 0,545 |
| **cN+ (TNM)** | - | 0,258 |
| **Portal ligature** | - | 0,192 |
| **Type of resection** | | |
| **Primary tumor** | - | 0,305 |
| **Metastasis** | - | 0,413 |
| **Number of resections** | - | 0,218 |
| **Clamping** | - | **0,025** |
| **Operating time** | - | 0,344 |
| **Incidents (Oslo)** | - | 0,404 |
| **Intraoperative transfusion** | - | 0,455 |
| **Conversion** | **8,571** | 0,121 |
| **Post-operative stay** | - | **0,006** |

### *c) Severe morbidity Clavien III, IV :*

**Table 75** Univariate analysis for severe morbidity.

| **Variable** | **Hazard ratio** | ***p*** |
|---|---|---|
| **Gender** | 1,375 | 0,676 |
| **Age (≤65 />65)** | - | 0,521 |
| **BMI (<25/≥25)** | 1,375 | 0,676 |
| **ASA comorbidities** | - | 0,174 |
| **History of abdominal surgery** | 2,167 | 0,550 |
| **Primitive (colon/rectum)** | 1,533 | 0,646 |
| **Anemia symptom** | - | 0,719 |
| **Unilobar/bilobar** | - | 0,521 |
| **Single/multiple** | 0,727 | 0,676 |
| **Size of metastasis** | | 0,643 |

| | | |
|---|---|---|
| All laparoscopic | - | 0,808 |
| Hybrid surgery | - | 0,354 |
| Down staging surgery | | 0,596 |
| Neoadjuvant treatment | - | 0,719 |
| Preoperative chemotherapy | - | 0,521 |
| Number of chemotherapy treatments | - | **0,008** |
| Preoperative radiotherapy | - | 0,558 |
| Hemoglobin < 10 g/dl | - | 0,763 |
| Albumin level (<35/≥35) | - | 0,636 |
| cT (TNM) | - | 0,854 |
| CN+ (TNM) | | 0,763 |
| Intraoperative transfusion | | 0,854 |
| Tumor differentiation on biopsy | - | 0,671 |
| N+ | | |
| Portal ligature | - | 0,719 |
| Type of resection | | |
| Primary tumor | - | 0,057 |
| Metastasis | - | 0,926 |
| Number of resections | | 0,212 |
| Clamping | - | 0,085 |
| Operating time | - | 0,988 |
| Intraoperative incidents (Oslo) | - | **0,010** |
| Conversion | - | 0,854 |
| Post-operative stay | - | **0,020** |
| Stay in intensive care | - | **0,036** |
| Number of days in intensive care | - | **0,020** |

### *d) Recidivism:*

**Table 76** Univariate analysis for recurrence.

| Variable | Hazard ratio | *p* |
|---|---|---|
| Gender | 0,607 | 0,406 |
| Age (≤65 />65) | 0,698 | 0,523 |
| BMI (<25/≥25) | 0,607 | 0,406 |
| ASA comorbidities | 1,979 | 0,301 |
| Previous abdominal surgery | 1,270 | 0,624 |
| High ACE rate | 2,528 | 0,251 |
| High 19.9 CA rate | 1,714 | 0,399 |
| Primitive (colon/rectum) | 0,692 | 0,475 |
| Location of metastasis | | 0,214 |

| | | |
|---|---|---|
| **Metastasis (single/multiple)** | 0,903 | 0,594 |
| **Unilobar/bilobar** | 2,743 | 0,190 |
| **Metastasis size** | - | 0,323 |
| **All laparoscopic** | 1,167 | 0,656 |
| **Hybrid surgery** | 0,789 | 0,525 |
| **Down staging surgery** | 2,083 | 0,320 |
| **Neoadjuvant treatment** | 0,519 | 0,410 |
| **Preoperative chemotherapy** | 0,696 | 0,477 |
| **Number of chemotherapy treatments** | - | 0,542 |
| **Preoperative radiotherapy** | 0,821 | 0,601 |
| **Tumor differentiation on biopsy** | - | 0,716 |
| **cT (TNM)** | 0,552 | 0,545 |
| **cN+ (TNM)** | **7,250** | **0,032** |
| **Portal ligature** | 1,929 | 0,410 |
| **Type of resection** | | |
| **Primary tumor** | - | 0,499 |
| **Metastasis** | - | 0,211 |
| **Number of resections** | - | 0,609 |
| **Operating time** | - | 0,612 |
| **Incidents (Oslo)** | - | 0,733 |
| **Intraoperative transfusion** | - | 0,455 |
| **Size of primary tumor** | - | 0,749 |
| **Histological type** | - | 0,278 |
| **R0 / R1 resection** | 0,625 | 0,575 |
| **pT (TNM)** | | 0,365 |
| **pN+ (TNM)** | **4,250** | 0,088 |
| **Conversion** | 0,757 | 0,455 |
| **Morbidity** | 0,689 | 0,523 |
| **Anastomotic fistula** | 3,750 | 0,404 |

## 14. Multivariate analysis :

Multivariate analysis to identify the factors that influenced morbidity in our series was performed using a Cox regression model after grouping variables whose *p* value was $\leq 0.05$ in univariate analysis.

### *a) For overall morbidity :*

**Table 77** Multivariate analysis of overall morbidity.

| Variable | Univariate analysis (*p* value) | Multivariate analysis (*p* value) |
|---|---|---|

| Anemia | 0,039 | **0,046** |
|---|---|---|
| Neoadjuvant treatment | 0,039 | 0,755 |
| Preoperative chemotherapy | 0,027 | 0,065 |
| Intraoperative incidents | 0,045 | 0,141 |
| Number of resections | 0,035 | **0,018** |

### *b) For mild morbidity :*

**Table 78** Multivariate analysis for mild morbidity.

| Variable | Univariate analysis (*p* value) | Multivariate analysis (*p* value) |
|---|---|---|
| Anemia | 0,016 | 0,120 |
| Neoadjuvant treatment | 0,016 | 0,599 |
| Preoperative chemotherapy | 0,007 | 0,079 |
| Clamping | 0,025 | 0,997 |
| Post-operative stay | 0,006 | **0,041** |

### *c) For severe morbidity :*

**Table 79** Multivariate analysis for severe morbidity.

| Variable | Univariate analysis (*p* value) | Multivariate analysis (*p* value) |
|---|---|---|
| Number of preoperative treatments | 0,008 | 0,996 |
| Intraoperative incidents | 0,010 | 0,998 |
| Stay in intensive care | 0,036 | 0,997 |
| Number of days in intensive care | 0,020 | 0,997 |

## B. Control arm :

### 1. Comparative study :

During the same period of our study, 74 patients were treated laparoscopically in our department for colorectal resection alone (without any associated liver procedure). We selected 40 of these patients on the basis of the following criteria:

Inclusion criteria:

1. Age > 18 years and < 80 years.
2. resectable adenocarcinoma of the rectum or colon.
3. Normal haematological, hepatic and renal tests.
4. Karnofsky index ≥ 70, WHO performance index ≤ 2.
5. informed consent.
6. Operated by the same surgeon (on the experimental arm).

Thirty-four patients were excluded because they did not meet the age criteria, or had been operated on by another surgeon, or on definitive anatomopathological study were not adenocarcinoma.

#### *a) General characteristics of the laparoscopic colorectal surgery arm alone :*

**Table 80** general characteristics of the control arm.

| | **Laparoscopic colorectal surgery = 40** |
|---|---|
| **Gender (M/F)** | 17/23 |
| **Age** | 60,28 ± 13,6 |
| **BMI** | 24,83 ± 3,99 |
| **ASA grade** | |
| **ASA I** | 19 (47,5) |
| **ASA II** | 20 (50) |
| **ASA III** | 01 (2,5) |
| **Tumor location** | |
| **Rectum** | 25 (62,5) |
| **Sigmoid** | 11 (27,5) |
| **Left colon** | 01 (2,5) |
| **Right colon** | 03 (7,5) |
| **Neoadjuvant radiotherapy** | 18 (45) |
| **Type of resection** | |
| **Anterior resection** | 21 (52,5) |
| **Segmental resection** | 09 (22,5) |

| | |
|---|---|
| **Abdominoperineal amputation** | 03 (7,5) |
| **Hartmann's intervention** | 02 (5) |
| **Right colectomy** | 03 (7,5) |
| **Subtotal colectomy** | 02 (5) |
| **TNM** | |
| **T1** | 1 (2,5) |
| **T2** | 4 (10) |
| **T3** | 35 (87,5) |
| **N+** | 36 (90) |

### *b) Surgical outcomes in the laparoscopic colorectal surgery alone arm*

**Table 81** Results of surgery in the control arm.

| | **laparoscopic colorectal surgery = 40** |
|---|---|
| **Operating time** | 274 ± 63.62 mn |
| **Conversion** | 4 (10) |
| **Clavien I II** | 9 (22,5) |
| **Clavien III IV** | 4(10) |
| **Anastomotic fistula** | 4(10) |
| **Post-operative stay** | 5,48 ± 2,81 |
| **Intraoperative transfusion** | 0 |
| **Mortality** | 0 |

### *c) Comparison of the population in the two study arms :*

**Table 82** Characteristics of patients and surgery in both arms.

| | **Control arm = 40** | **Experimental arm = 40** | ***p* value** |
|---|---|---|---|
| **Gender (M/F)** | 17/23 | 23/17 | 0,132 |
| **Age** | 60,28 ± 13,6 | 59,08 ± 11,28 | 0,669 |
| **BMI** | 24,83 ± 3,99 | 24,05 ± 4,06 | 0,392 |
| **ASA grade** | | | 0,490 |
| **ASA I** | 19 (47,5) | 23 (57,5) | |
| **ASA II** | 20 (50) | 15 (37,5) | |
| **ASA III** | 01 (2,5) | 02 (5) | |
| **Tumor location** | | | 0,184 |
| **Rectum** | 25 (62,5) | 16 (40) | |
| **Sigmoid** | 11 (27,5) | 16 (40) | |

| | | | |
|---|---|---|---|
| **Left colon** | 01 (2,5) | 4 (10) | |
| **Right colon** | 03 (7,5) | 4 (10) | |
| **Neoadjuvant radiotherapy** | 18 (45) | 10 (25) | 0,061 |
| **Type of resection** | | | 0,221 |
| **Anterior resection** | 21 (52,5) | 14 (35) | |
| **Segmental resection** | 09 (22,5) | 13 (32,5) | |
| **Abdominoperineal** | 03 (7,5) | 02 (5) | |
| **amputation** | 02 (5) | 00 (0) | |
| **Hartmann's intervention** | 03 (7,5) | 04 (10) | |
| **Right colectomy** | 00 (00) | 04 (10) | |
| **Left colectomy** | 02 (5) | 02 (5) | |
| **Subtotal colectomy** | 00 (00) | 01 (2,5) | |
| **Total colectomy** | | | |
| **TNM** | | | 0,549 |
| **T1** | 1 (2,5) | 0 (0) | |
| **T2** | 4 (10) | 3 (7,5) | |
| **T3** | 35 (87,5) | 37 (92,5) | |
| **N+** | 36 (90) | 35 (87,5) | 0,500 |

**Table 83** Comparison of surgical results in the two arms.

| | **Control arm = 40** | **Experimental arm = 40** | ***p* value** |
|---|---|---|---|
| **Operating time** | 274 ± 63.62 mn | 323 ± 52,6 | < 0.0005 |
| **Conversion** | 4 (10) | 3 (7,5) | 0,500 |
| **Overall morbidity** | 13 (32,5) | 11 (27,5) | 0,606 |
| **Clavien I II** | 9 (22,5) | 9 (22,5) | 1,000 |
| **Clavien III IV** | 4(10) | 2 (5) | 0,338 |
| **Anastomotic fistula** | 4(10) | 2 (5) | 0,338 |
| **Intraoperative transfusion** | 0 (0) | 3 (7,5) | 0,120 |
| **Post-operative stay** | 5,48 ± 2,81 | 5,10 ± 2,58 | 0,537 |

### *d) Overall morbidity factors in both arms of the study N=80 :*

Multivariate analysis of factors predictive of overall morbidity in the entire study population, including both arms.

**Table 84** Multivariate analysis of overall morbidity in both arms.

| **Variable** | **Multivariate analysis (*p* value)** |
|---|---|
| **Female gender** | **0,016** |
| **Age > 65** | **0,045** |
| **Post-operative stay** | **0,006** |

## C. Summary of results :

During the 41 months of our study, two arms were set up.
An experimental arm called the simultaneous laparoscopic surgery arm, and a control arm called the colorectal laparoscopic surgery alone arm.
In the experimental arm, 50 patients met the inclusion criteria. Ten patients were excluded secondarily, so the analysis was based on 40 patients.
In the control arm, 40 patients met the inclusion criteria.
In the experimental arm, the mean age was 59.08 years, with a sex ratio of 1.35. The primary tumor was colonic in 60% of cases and rectal in 40%. MH was unique in 42.5% of patients. Hybrid surgery was performed in 60% of patients, down-staging surgery in 22.5% and totally laparoscopic surgery in 10%. The conversion rate was 7.5%. Factors associated with conversion were the degree of severity of the intraoperative incident according to the grades of the Oslo classification ($p$ = 0.044) and the degree of parietal infiltration on anatomopathological study ($p$ = 0.011).
Mean operating time was 323 min for the complete procedure, 221.8 min for the colorectal section and 101.2 min for the liver section. Operating time for hybrid surgery was longer than for other procedures ($p$ = 0.017). The duration of down-staging surgery was the shortest among the different procedures ($p$ = 0.041).
After portal ligation, 5/6 patients had significantly enlarged the remaining future liver, with a mean gain in volume of 59.48%.
Major hepatectomy was subsequently performed in all 6 patients (no drop-out).
An intraoperative incident occurred in 25% of patients (Oslo Grade 1 in 10%, Oslo Grade 2 in 15%). The occurrence of an intraoperative incident was statistically linked to the presence of comorbidities ($p$ = 0.049). The occurrence of a severe incident (Oslo 2) was linked to previous abdominal surgery, especially if the anterior incision was a midline incision ($p$ = 0.013).
For the primary tumour, 95% of resections were R0. For resection of liver metastases, the R0 resection rate was 92.8% in relation to the number of parts analyzed, and 90% in relation to the number of patients.
The mean number of nodes removed in the curage was 15.55. Patients who had received chemotherapy preoperatively had significantly fewer nodes removed (13.31 vs. 21.45) ($p$ = 0.034).
Overall morbidity at 30 days was 27.5%, represented mainly by mild morbidity in 22.5% of the entire study population, and 81.82% of patients with a complication. In multivariate analysis alone, anemia ($p$ = 0.046) and the number of liver resections ($p$ = 0.018) were independent factors in morbidity.
Postoperative mortality at 30 days was nil.
Postoperative hospital stay averaged 5.1 ± 2.58 days.

Patient follow-up averaged 15 months, with a median of 12.5 months and extremes ranging from 2 months to 41 months.
During this period, 9 patients had a recurrence (22.5%), with a mean time to recurrence of 13.55 months.
All patients in our study were alive at the time of point.
Mean recurrence-free survival was 28.91 months. Median recurrence-free survival was 27 months. Only one variable was associated with recurrence: N+ cTNM classification ($p = 0.032$).
The populations of the two arms were comparable according to the following variables: age, gender, ASA grade, neoadjuvant radiotherapy, primary tumor location, type of colorectal resection and T and N stage of the primary tumor.
There was no difference between the two groups in overall morbidity ($p = 0.606$), mild morbidity ($p = 1.000$) and severe morbidity ($p = 0.338$).
Analysis of morbidity risk factors for the entire population (both arms) did not find that belonging to one group or the other influenced the occurrence of more complications.
Between the two arms, there was no difference in conversion rate ($p = 0.500$), fistula rate ($p = 0.338$), intraoperative transfusion rate ($p = 0.120$) and postoperative stay ($p = 0.537$).
Operating time was longer in the simultaneous surgery arm, with a highly significant difference ($p < 0.0005$).

# VIII. Discussion:

## A. Epidemiology and patient characteristics:

In our series, the most affected age group was 60-70 years, with 18 patients (45% of the total), and a median age of 62.5 years (32-79 years). It should be noted that 3 patients (7.5% of the total) were under 40 years of age, i.e. metastatic at a young age, which testifies to the aggressiveness of the disease.
The sex ratio was 1.35 (predominantly male).
S.Ferretti (35) in the largest multicenter series published to date, on the results of the simultaneous laparoscopic approach in the management of colorectal cancer with synchronous liver metastases, included 142 patients, with a median age of 66 (32 - 85) and a sex ratio of 0.86 (predominantly female). Garritano (37) in his systematic review of this minimally invasive approach, included 150 patients from 20 different publications, with a median age of 60 (31 - 88), but did not report the sex of the patients.
Lupinacci (34) in his systematic review which preceded Garritano's, reported a population of 39 patients, without giving demographic details. In his metanalysis, Chen (14) who compared strategies (simultaneous and sequential) in the management of CCRMHS, reported the demographic results of 14 studies including 2204 metastatic patients, which are summarized in the following table:

**Table 85** Median age of patients included in the metanalysis by Chen et al. (14).

| First author | Year | Country | Study type | Simultaneous resection | | Staged resection | | Quality score |
|---|---|---|---|---|---|---|---|---|
| | | | | Patients | Age | Patients | Age | |
| Capussotti et al. | 2007 | Italy | Retro | 70 | 64.9 | 57 | 60 | 8 |
| Chua et al. | 2004 | America | Retro | 64 | 63 | 32 | 61 | 8 |
| Jaeck et al. | 1999 | France | Retro | 28 | 56 | 31 | 60 | 6 |
| Martin et al. | 2003 | America | Retro | 134 | 64 | 106 | 61 | 8 |
| Martin et al. | 2009 | America | Retro | 70 | 58 | 160 | 61 | 8 |
| Reddy et al. | 2007 | America | Retro | 135 | 57 | 475 | 58 | 8 |
| Slupski et al. | 2009 | Poland | Retro | 28 | 59.4 | 61 | 60.2 | 7 |
| Tanaka et al. | 2004 | Japan | Retro | 39 | 64 | 37 | 65 | 8 |
| Thelen et al. | 2007 | German | Retro | 40 | 60.5 | 179 | 59.7 | 7 |
| Turrini et al. | 2007 | France | Retro | 57 | 60 | 62 | 59 | 9 |
| Vassiliou et al. | 2007 | Greece | Retro | 25 | 63 | 78 | 61 | 7 |
| Vogt et al. | 1991 | German | Retro | 19 | NR | 17 | NR | 6 |
| Weber et al. | 2003 | France | Retro | 35 | 58 | 62 | 60 | 8 |
| Yan et al. | 2007 | Australia | Retro | 73 | 60 | 30 | 59 | 8 |

*Retro* retrospective, *NR* not recorded

The median age in these studies ranged from 56 to 65.
More than half (57.5%) of our patients had no comorbidities and were classified as ASA I by the American Society of Anesthesiologists. All were in good general condition at inclusion, and were classified as 0 according to the WHO performance status.

Among patients with comorbidities, arterial hypertension (AH) was present 10 times and diabetes 9 times, and these two pathologies were associated in 7 patients.
Two terrain-related factors could influence the difficulty of our laparoscopic surgical approach, high BMI and a history of abdominal surgery.
Seventeen patients (42.5%) were overweight (BMI ≥ 25), while 3 patients (7.5%) were obese (BMI ≥ 30).
After statistical analysis, high BMI was not a risk factor for morbidity ($p = 0.305$) or conversion ($p = 0.260$) in our series.
Previous abdominal surgery was not a factor in morbidity ($p = 0.514$).
Twelve patients, or 30% of our series, had a history of abdominal surgery, which we did not consider a contraindication to the laparoscopic approach.
The extent of postoperative adhesions caused by the first operation was in fact related to the type of surgery, so if there was a history of laparoscopic cholecystectomy, appendectomy via a McBurney route or colostomy via an elective route, our laparoscopic approach was almost equivalent to an approach to a virgin abdomen, as adhesions were so few, on the other hand, in the case of a previous median incision (a fortiori xypho-pubic), caution was called for when introducing the first trocar (open laparoscopy), as additional laparoscopic adhesiolysis time was required, with the risk of visceral lesions (see video 2). The occurrence of a severe incident, grade 2 of the Oslo classification, was statistically correlated ($p = 0.013$) with previous midline incision, whereas previous abdominal surgery was not a risk factor for intraoperative incident ($p = 0.095$) or conversion ($p = 0.704$).

## B. Diagnosis:

### 1. Clinical :

In our series, the presenting signs were related to the primary tumour and not to hepatic metastatic disease. Clinical signs related to hepatic extension are often delayed and reflect unresectable metastases.
All our patients were symptomatic; no patient was included after a screening diagnosis.
Symptoms began on average 4.6 ± 2.4 months before diagnosis, with the most frequent symptoms being rectal discharge and transit disorders.
Anemia was indicative of the disease in 10% of patients and had a negative impact on overall morbidity (poor prognostic factor) ($p = 0.001$).
No patient was rejected for surgery or laparoscopic approach on physical examination, because of, for example, distant extension (Troisier lymph node), ascites, fixed abdominal mass, altered general condition WHO ≥ 2, large ventration...

### 2. Low endoscopy:

It was systematically combined with biopsy, and led to the diagnosis of primary colorectal cancer in all cases. (52).

Total colonoscopy was possible (non-stenosing tumor) in 22 patients.
In the case of impassable stenosing tumors, colonoscopy was systematically performed postoperatively, while colonoscopy was performed in only 10 patients preoperatively, and did not reveal synchronous lesions in all cases.

## 3. Imaging:

In the case of a primary rectal tumor, pelvic MRI was systematically included in the local and locoregional extension workup, in addition to digital rectal examination. Endorectal ultrasonography has not been included in the extension workup for rectal tumors, as this examination is intended for small tumors in order to differentiate T1 and T2 tumors, and also for the evaluation of T1 tumors prior to local excision (129). In our series, 87.5% of rectal tumours were classified as T3.
Pelvic MRI was used to localize the tumor, perform T and N staging, and specify the circumferential resection margin and sphincter relationships.
False-positive lesions were noted on five occasions, on CT three times (angiomatous lesions after anatomopathological study, initially described as hepatic metastases and which were associated with other metastatic lesions without consequence on management) and on MRI twice (lesions initially described as metastatic, then as cystic lesions on re-evaluation after completion of neoadjuvant treatment), which led us to change the therapeutic strategy (laparoscopic surgery of the primary tumor alone). These two patients were excluded from the study. Subsequent monitoring of the lesions confirmed their cystic nature.
In the literature, the sensitivity and specificity of the various morphological examinations in detecting liver metastases have been evaluated: Floriani et al. (130) after a review of 6030 articles and an evaluation of 25 specific studies, estimated the sensitivity of ultrasound at 63 - 97.6%, CT at 74.8 - 95.6%, MRI at 81.1 - 97.2% and FDG-PET at 93.8 - 98.7%.
The specificity of ultrasound was 97.6% (95.6-99.5), CT 95.6% (93.4-97.8), MRI 97.2% (94.5-99.9) and FDG-PET 98.7% (97.2-100).
In practice, CT TAP was performed routinely, while liver MRI was performed on request.
PET scan provides important information, particularly on intra-abdominal and extrahepatic metastases (52). Its indication should be discussed in the PCR.
We requested it in a single patient presenting with a suspected recurrence in the form of a single peritoneal nodule on PET scan. The PET scan had confirmed the metastatic nature of this single nodule, with no other localizations elsewhere. The nodule (epiploic implant) was resected laparoscopically, and the diagnosis was confirmed on pathological anatomy.

## 4. Biology:

The preoperative laboratory work-up had detected a hemoglobin level (Hb < 10 g/dl) in 5 patients (12.5%), a disturbance of the liver balance in two patients (5%) (mild cytolysis in one patient, anicteric cholestasis in another) who had received neoadjuvant chemotherapy.
All patients had a normal blood count.

Blood glucose levels were > 1.40 g/l in 5 of the 10 diabetic patients in the series. Glycated hemoglobin was elevated in two patients despite correct blood glucose levels.
Albumin levels were <35 g/l in 7 patients (17.5%).
In each case, the data from the biological workup were used to guide the measures to be taken to prepare the patients, in coordination with the intensive care physicians (decision on preoperative transfusion, iron injection, administration of albumin, initiation of regular insulin, etc.).
Biological tests carried out preoperatively could also form part of the disease assessment, as in the case of the tumor markers ACE and CA 19.9, which are systematically requested before the start of treatment and during postoperative monitoring.
CEA levels were elevated (> 5µg/l) in 25 patients (62.5%), CA 19.9 levels were elevated (> 37 U/l) in 10 patients (25%), and a combination of elevated levels of both markers was found in 9 patients.
These findings lead us to question the CA 19.9 assay, since virtually every time CA 19.9 levels are elevated, CEA levels are also elevated, although the reverse is not true.
All the more so since, in the TNCD 2019 recommendations (52) the ACE assay is a grade C recommendation without mentioning the CA 19.9 assay.

## C. Strategy:

The poor long-term survival results of MHSCCR patients managed according to a conventional strategy had led to questions about the timing and sequence of possible therapeutic interventions. Currently, there are four possible therapeutic strategies:
(1) The primary approach to the primary tumor (classic approach), which involves resection of the primary colorectal tumor followed by chemotherapy, with subsequent liver resection performed 3-6 months after colorectal resection (provided that liver metastases are still resectable).
(2) Simultaneous resection of the primary colorectal tumor and liver metastases in a single procedure (combined approach) for selected patients.
(3) Liver first ″liver first″ (or chemotherapy first) this approach comprises preoperative chemotherapy (3-6 cycles) followed by liver resection, then chemotherapy in the interim followed by resection of the primary colorectal tumor (it is suitable for patients with asymptomatic primary tumor and initially potentially resectable liver metastases).
(4) Up-front hepatectomy, which involves initial liver resection followed by interval chemotherapy, then colorectal resection followed by chemotherapy. (This strategy can be offered to patients with an asymptomatic primary tumor and initially resectable liver metastases).

The rationale behind the primary approach is twofold: primary colorectal tumors are seen as a likely source of subsequent metastases, and also as the source of symptoms. The main advantage of this strategy is to avoid potential complications

associated with the primary tumor, and to reduce the risk of potential colorectal tumor progression during a reverse approach (liver surgery or initial chemotherapy). Conversely, the main drawback of this approach is the risk of progression of liver metastases that may become unresectable in the interim after resection of the primary tumor (particularly in patients who have experienced a postoperative complication after colorectal resection).
Due to the frequent progression of liver metastases, only a few patients benefit from the classic sequential strategy. In 2012, an analysis based on LiverMetSurvey revealed that less than 30% of patients followed the complete treatment plan of the colorectal tumor-first strategy (from primary tumor resection to liver resection) (131). Conversely, the reverse strategy enables completion of the treatment plan in almost 80% of patients (132).

The strategy of simultaneous resection has been proposed to avoid delaying surgical resection of metastatic liver disease. The main advantage of this strategy is the removal of both tumour sites in a single operation, followed by systemic chemotherapy with minimal delay. Conversely, the main disadvantage of this strategy is the risk of increased postoperative morbidity and possibly mortality. Risk of infectious liver complications (due to bacterial contamination from the colorectal resection), risk of anastomotic complications (due to impaired liver function).
Several studies have demonstrated that a reasonable morbidity/mortality rate can be achieved if colorectal resection is combined with minor hepatectomy. In a systematic review evaluating simultaneous resections in several series, postoperative morbidity ranged from 5% to 48% when minor hepatectomies were performed, and from 33% to 55% when major hepatectomies were performed (133).
Simultaneous resection is best suited to selected patients; many authors recommend considering simultaneous resection only if one of the two surgical resections is minor. It is reasonable to perform a rectal resection simultaneously with a minor hepatectomy (<3 segments), or to perform liver resections (≥ 3 segments) simultaneously with a right colon resection. However, hepatectomies should only be performed by an experienced hepatobiliary team. Patients' general state of health and comorbidities must be taken into consideration (134).

Liver first (or chemotherapy first), this reverse treatment strategy was first introduced by Mentha et al in 2008 (132). It comprises initial preoperative chemotherapy (3-6 cycles) followed by liver resection and then resection of the primary colorectal tumor.
The prognosis of patients with stage IV colorectal cancer is determined primarily by the curability of liver metastases, and not by the primary tumor or its potential complications.
The advantages of the chemotherapy-first approach are: early application of systemic therapy; reduced risk of progression of liver metastases; and the possibility of downsizing liver metastases or, better still, converting unresectable liver metastases to resectable status.

Since stage IV colorectal cancer presents as a systemic disease, it seems reasonable to offer chemotherapy as soon as possible after the diagnosis has been made. Moreover, patients with synchronous liver metastases are thought to have more aggressive tumors with less favorable cancer biology.
By using chemotherapy initially, effective systemic treatment is not delayed by colorectal surgery and its possible post-operative complications.
In theory, another possible benefit of preoperative chemotherapy is the elimination of micrometastatic disease and the eradication of dormant cancer cells.
The reverse strategy is best suited to patients with an asymptomatic primary tumor and advanced liver metastatic disease.
Up-front hepatectomy: the common sequence of the initial hepatectomy strategy includes liver resection, interval chemotherapy, colorectal resection followed by adjuvant chemotherapy. This strategy was initially proposed by Grundmann et al in 2008 for patients with asymptomatic colorectal tumor and resectable synchronous liver metastases (134).
This strategy would avoid the main drawbacks of preoperative chemotherapy, including liver toxicity, missing lesions (missing metastases) and the risk of tumor progression. In addition, chemotherapy increases the risk of systemic toxicity, postoperative bleeding and infection (by inducing neutropenia).

The choice of one or other of these strategies in colorectal cancer patients with synchronous liver metastases depends on several parameters, including the patient's performance status, comorbidities and tumor stage. An individual treatment plan needs to be drawn up for each patient in a multidisciplinary concertation meeting that includes experienced colorectal and hepatobiliary surgeons.
The classic strategy (primary approach to the primary tumor) is best suited to patients with a symptomatic primary tumor and synchronous liver metastases.
Evaluation of the feasibility of the simultaneous approach should be reserved for patients with limited extent of hepatic metastatic disease, when a minor resection procedure is envisaged.
For patients with unresectable or borderline resectable metastases, the primary chemotherapy approach should be preferred.
For patients with resectable metastases, the Up-front hepatectomy approach is feasible.

None of the above treatment strategies appears to be inferior to the others (135). However, the optimal therapeutic strategy is still unclear due to the limited amount of evidence. It is necessary to create an individual treatment plan for each patient with synchronous liver metastases in multidisciplinary consultation meetings, evaluating all strategies with the aim of avoiding unnecessary surgical complications and improving prognosis.

In the early 1990s, simultaneous surgery was considered to be associated with greater morbidity and poorer prognosis than sequential surgery (15).

The publication of more recent series had shown that the simultaneous approach was feasible and safe, and had the same short- and long-term results compared with sequential surgery on selected patients (136,137) .

This prompted authors to compare the two strategies on larger patient populations, notably Chen's metanalysis (14) which included 2204 patients from 14 comparative publications, the simultaneous approach had the advantage (significant difference) of a shorter hospital stay and reduced morbidity. Survival rates at 1, 3 and 5 years did not differ from the sequential surgery group.

He concluded that the simultaneous approach was the approach of choice in selected patients. This selection of patients by the authors when choosing the strategy was considered a bias in the interpretation of the results of this metanalysis, especially as there were no randomized studies included in this analysis; all 14 studies were retrospective. Patients eligible for simultaneous surgery were the ″least severe″ in terms of liver metastatic disease.

Another meta-analysis published more recently by Li (138)which included 2,724 patients from 19 comparative (non-randomized) studies, reached the same conclusions as the previous one, with shorter hospital stays and lower morbidity for simultaneous surgery. Survival at 1, 3 and 5 years was similar in both groups. There was no difference between the two groups in terms of mortality, blood loss or recurrence rate. However, the author pointed to the same selection bias in the simultaneous surgery group.

We understand that simultaneous surgery is intended for selected patients, to achieve the good results reported in the literature.

One element of selection is the extent of planned liver resection, since Reddy et al. (21) in a multi-institutional analysis showed that, compared with a sequential approach, synchronous resection resulted in shorter hospital stays and lower morbidity for minor hepatectomies, but morbidity was higher when major hepatectomies were performed (36.1% vs. 17.6%).

Simultaneous surgery therefore appears to be of interest for patients who do not require major liver resection, and who have an uncomplicated primary colorectal tumor.

The aim of our study was to evaluate laparoscopic surgery in the management of MHSCCR using a combined strategy, to do so among the patient selection criteria was the planned minor extent of liver resection.

Our patients were eligible for simultaneous or down-staging surgery, both in terms of general condition, since all were WHO 0, and in terms of their comorbidities, which were controlled.

Although all patients in our series were candidates for combined surgery, the therapeutic sequence was established on a case-by-case basis.

Several sequences were possible, depending on the location of the primary tumor (colon or rectum), the resectable or potentially resectable nature of the liver metastases and their extent, even leading to discussion of two-stage surgery (performed on 9 patients in the series).

The location of the primary tumor was an important factor in the decision-making process, since 10 of the 16 patients with rectal tumors had an indication for neoadjuvant radiotherapy. Neoadjuvant treatment in the metastatic setting should not delay management of secondary hepatic localization, which is why we favored a short radiotherapy protocol with immediate surgery whenever possible. The short protocol was administered in 8 patients (80%), and surgery was immediate in 5. Surgery was deferred in three patients for various reasons:

- Toxicity of chemotherapy given just before radiotherapy.
- Delay in prescribing an anti-angiogenic agent (Bevacizumab) just prior to radiotherapy.
- Organizational.

Deferring surgery in these three patients was not deleterious, since at re-evaluation there had been no progression of metastases, in initially limited hepatic metastatic disease (single nodule in two patients, two nodules in one patient).
Two patients had undergone CCR for tumors of the middle and lower rectum associated with a single small metastasis that was immediately resectable.

The non-symptomatic nature of the primary tumor was an important criterion in the choice of the combined strategy. Nevertheless, in our series, 4 patients had presented with an occlusive syndrome during chemotherapy and had undergone emergency surgery, with a near-abdominal colostomy performed on each occasion (twice via the median route and twice via the elective route); this abdominal procedure was not considered a contraindication to our subsequent laparoscopic approach during the resection procedure.

The second decision-making factor was the classification of liver metastases, their number, size and location.
In the case of resectable metastases, perioperative chemotherapy was given prior to surgery, and in the case of rectal tumors, this chemotherapy shortly preceded radiotherapy.
In the case of a single small metastasis < 2 cm, surgery was performed immediately or after radiotherapy if the latter was indicated.
In the case of potentially resectable metastases, the addition of targeted therapy to chemotherapy was based on RAS status. Eighteen patients had received targeted therapy prior to surgery, of whom 11 had received an anti-angiogenic and 7 an anti-EGFR.
In the case of bilobar metastases and when a two-stage hepatectomy was decided, chemotherapy combined with targeted therapy was started, followed by a first surgical stage known as "down staging", combining resection of the primary tumor with a hepatic stage that could be either a resection procedure alone, portal ligation alone or a combination of both.
A second hepatic period was scheduled a few weeks later, either to wait for liver hypertrophy or simply for rehabilitation. During this waiting period, chemotherapy was administered.

The third decision-making factor was the patient's general condition, which was regularly reassessed during oncology, surgery or anesthesia consultations.
We had deferred surgery in a patient presenting with a rectal tumor with a single segment III liver metastasis, after short radiotherapy, for altered general condition and biological disturbances.
Table 86 summarizes the various therapeutic sequences adopted in our patients.

**Table 86** The different therapeutic sequences.

| Therapeutic sequence | Number | Percentage |
|---|---|---|
| **Initial surgery** | 06 | 15% |
| **CT+TC then surgery** | 17 | 42,5% |
| **Perioperative CT followed by surgery** | 07 | 17,5% |
| **CT then short RT then immediate surgery** | 03 | 7,5% |
| **Short RT followed by immediate surgery** | 02 | 5% |
| **CCR then delayed surgery** | 02 | 5% |
| **CT+TC then short RT then deferred surgery** | 01 | 2,5% |
| **CT then short RT then deferred surgery** | 01 | 2,5% |
| **Short RT followed by delayed surgery** | 01 | 2,5% |
| **Total** | 40 | 100 % |

## D. Approach:

One of the prerequisites for successful digestive surgery is good exposure of the operating field.
In conventional surgery, exposure depends on the type and length of the incision, the patient's morphotype and the use of retractors and valves.

In colorectal surgery, wide midline incisions are often necessary, as the procedure involves different abdominal compartments, sometimes far from the tumor site (e.g. mobilization of the left colonic angle for resection of a rectal tumor). These midline incisions are not without early or late morbidities. Some examples include reduced respiratory capacity in the immediate postoperative period, and the risk of evisceration and ventration.
In liver surgery, on the other hand, transverse incisions are preferred, notably under the right rib or bisous-costal.
A combined inverted-L incision, commonly known as the Makuuchi incision, gives a very good view of the entire liver region.
In combined surgery for colorectal cancer and synchronous liver metastases, choosing the right approach becomes an important step in the surgical strategy.
This choice will depend not only on the patient's morphotype (brevilinear, longilinear, BMI), but also on the topography not only of the primary tumour, but also of liver metastases (right liver/left liver, anterior segments/posterior segments).

At the extreme, a rectal tumour associated with hepatic metastases in the posterior segments in a patient with a short stature would require a long xypho-pubic incision associated with a right subcostal slit, or even more, for an adequate approach in conventional surgery (Fig. 53). This incision is very debilitating, with significant parietal trauma, and the action of the retractors and valves and their impact on postoperative pain and ventilatory mechanics.

The surgical community was not unanimous in its support for this unpleasant approach, and often preferred sequential surgery, which was intellectually more comfortable for the surgeon, since by deferring a surgical step he thought he was protecting the patient from a complication.

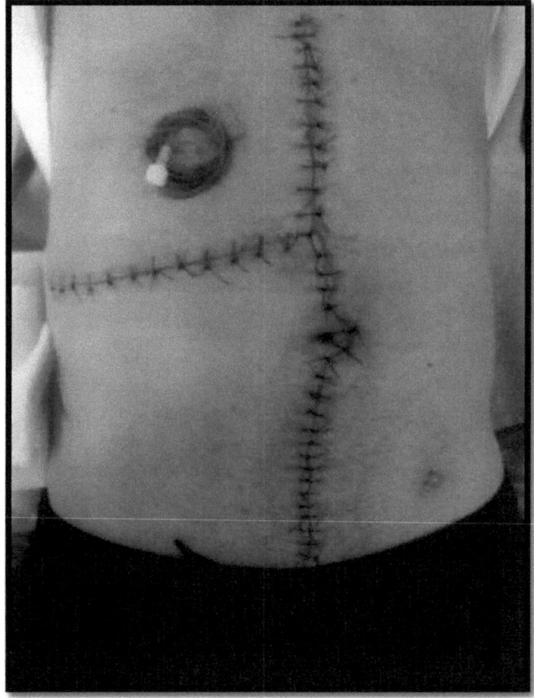

**Figure 53** Conventional approach for simultaneous surgery (CPMC).

But is there an alternative to this approach?

Laparoscopic surgery, also known as minimally invasive surgery, reduces aggression and surgical stress, as well as the inflammatory response to surgical trauma. It reduces postoperative pain. It also reduces the risk of parietal complications (sepsis, ventration). Transit and feeding are resumed more rapidly.

It improves patient rehabilitation, with a faster return to normal life, and consequently shortens hospital stays. Some laparoscopic surgical procedures are now performed on an outpatient basis. Time off work is shortened.
A reduction in the risk of infection has been noted. It also reduces postoperative adhesions.
On the other hand, for some procedures, the operating time may be shorter than for the conventional approach, while for others it may be longer. Finally, the aesthetic benefits are undeniable.
This new approach has been evaluated and compared with the conventional approach for numerous digestive surgery procedures, and has been validated for some of them, and is even considered a ″gold standard ″ for a few. (Cholecystectomy, Nissen, Heller...)
In colorectal surgery, laparoscopic surgery was initially introduced to perform colectomies for benign pathologies. The first laparoscopic colectomy was performed in 1991 by Jacobs (139).
Laparoscopic colon cancer surgery was initially hampered by the occurrence of trocar-port metastases (first described in 1993) (140). After this case was described, several small studies revealed an incidence of trocar-hole metastases of up to 21% (Table 87). However, this major problem of laparoscopy in malignancies has not been confirmed in more recent studies. These have reported a rate of trocar-port metastases of between 0% and 1.4% (Table 80), which is comparable to the rate of abdominal wall metastases after open surgery in two large retrospective studies involving over a thousand patients (0.6 and 0.8%) (141,142).

**Table 87** Incidence of trocar-port metastases after colectomy (143).

| Author | Year | N/total | % |
|---|---|---|---|
| **1993 - 1996** | | | |
| - Guillou | 1993 | 1/57 | 1,8 % |
| - Berends | 1994 | 4/14 | 21 % |
| - Drouard | 1995 | 12/507 | 2,4 % |
| - Boulez | 1996 | 3/117 | 2,5 % |
| **1997 - 2002** | | | |
| - Bouvet | 1998 | 0/91 | 0 % |
| - Leung | 1999 | 1/179 | 0,6 % |
| - Schiedeck | 1999 | 1/399 | 0,25 % |
| - Franklin | 2000 | 0/50 | 0 % |
| - Lujan | 2002 | 1/102 | 1 % |
| - Lezoche | 2002 | 2/140 | 1,4 % |
| - Anderson | 2002 | 1/100 | 1% |

| - Lechaux | 2002 | 1/206 | 0,5 % |
|---|---|---|---|
| - Lumley | 2002 | 1/181 | 0,6 % |
| - Lacy | 2002 | 1/106 | 0,9 % |

Apart from the advantages of laparoscopy in terms of rehabilitation quality and good short-term results, which have been verified in the literature, it was also necessary to demonstrate the carcinological efficacy of the technique, since in patients with cancer, carcinological prognosis takes precedence over functional prognosis. This assessment concerns the quality of excision, the recurrence rate and survival.

Since then, several randomized Phase III trials have been published, validating laparoscopic surgery for colon cancer.

The main studies are summarized in the following table:

**Table 88** Main phase III studies validating laparoscopic surgery for colon cancer (144).

| Variable | COLOR | COST | CLASICC* | LAPKON II | ALCCaS | Barcelona | Liang | LAFA-study† |
|---|---|---|---|---|---|---|---|---|
| Study design, Phase III | multi | multi | multi | multi | multi | single | single | multi |
| Concealment | Computer-generated random numbers | Centralized | Centralized by telephone | Centralized by telephone Revealed during operation | Centralized | Sealed envelopes | Random-sized blocks 2-10 | 2 × 2 Internet randomization module |
| Median follow-up, mo | 53 | 60 | 37 | § | § | 43 | 40 | — |
| Primary outcomes | 3-year DFS | Time to recurrence | 3-year DFS 3-year OS LR | § | § | Cancer-related survival | Time to recurrence | Total postop hospital stay |
| Level of evidence‡ | I | I | I | I | I | II | II | I |
| Population, no | | | | | | | | |
| OP | 542 | 428 | 140 | 222 | 298 | 102 | 134 | 108 |
| LAP | 534 | 435 | 273 | 250 | 294 | 106 | 135 | 110 |
| Tumour stage | | | | | | | | |
| I | 24% | 26% (OP) 35% (LAP) | NA | 28% (OP) 35% (LAP) | 23% | 22% | — | NA |
| II | 43% | 34% (OP) 31% (LAP) | NA | 38% (OP) 32% (LAP) | 40% | 43% | 49% | NA |
| III | 33% | 28% (OP) 26% (LAP) | NA | 33% (OP) 33% (LAP) | 30% | 35% | 51% | NA |
| IV | — | 4% (OP) 2% (LAP) | NA | — | 2% | — | — | NA |
| Postoperative chemotherapy | According to surgeon ($p = 0.99$) | According to surgeon | 29% (OP) 28% (LAP) | NA | NA | 56% (OP) 61% (LAP) | For stage III patients | NA |
| Surgery | | | | | | | | |
| Surgical procedure | | | | | | | | |
| Right | 47% | 54% | 45% | 29% | 58% | 45% | — | 48% |
| Left | 11% | 7% | 13% | ¶ | 4% | 2% | 70% | 49% |
| Sigmoid | 38% | 38% | 21% | ¶ | — | 45% | 30% | — |
| Anterior | — | — | 11% | — | 38% | 6% | — | — |
| Conversion rate | 19% | 21% | 25% | 11% | 15% | 11% | 3% | 11% |
| Surgeon experience | ≥ 20 LAP colectomies | ≥ 20 LAP colectomies | ≥ 20 LAP resections | ≥ 20 LAP colectomies | 52% surgeons treated > 10 patients | Experienced team | Experienced surgeon | ≥ 20 LAP for benign disease |

CLASICC = Conventional Versus Laparoscopic-Assisted Surgery in Patients with Colorectal Cancer; COLOR = Colon Cancer Laparoscopic or Open Resection; COST = Clinical Outcomes of Surgical Therapy; DFS = disease-free survival; LAP = laparoscopy; LR = local recurrence; multi = multicentred; NA = not available; OP = open surgery; OS = overall survival; single = single-centred.

*This trial included patients with colon and rectum cancers. When available, only data specific to colon cancer are presented.

†This trial evaluated fast-track versus standard care and LAP versus OP (4 arms). Only the 2 arms with standard care (LAP v. OP) are presented.

‡As evaluated according to the American Society of Clinical Oncology and European Society for Medical Oncology gradation system (see Table 1).

§Only short-term outcomes are published.

¶71% for left plus rectosigmoid.

Laparoscopic surgery for rectal cancer, considered advanced surgery, was validated much later, on the basis of randomized phase III trials (table 89), under certain conditions related to the tumor itself, since laparoscopy is recommended for T1, T2 and low T3 tumors, or to the surgical environment, since it must be reserved for expert centers.

**Table 89** Main phase III studies validating laparoscopic surgery for rectal cancer (144).

| Variable | Liang | COREAN | CLASICC* | Lujan | Ng | Ng | Pechlivanides | Braga* | Zhou |
|---|---|---|---|---|---|---|---|---|---|
| Study design, Phase III | single | multi | multi | single | single | single | multi | single | single |
| Concealment | Opaque envelopes | Computer-generated | Centralized, by phone | Computer-generated | Computer-generated | Computer-generated | Computer-generated | Computer-generated | NA |
| Median follow-up, mo. | 44 | NA | 37 | 34 (OP)<br>33 (LAP) | 113 (OP)<br>109 (LAP) | 91 (OP)<br>87 (LAP) | NA | 54 | NA |
| Primary outcomes | 3-year OS | DFS | 5-year DFS, 5-year OS, LR | No. lymph nodes retrieved, integrity of mesorectal resection margin | Long-term morbidity | Postoperative recovery | No. lymph nodes retrieved | Short-term postopmorbidity | Short-term results |
| Level of evidence† | I | I | I | I | I | I | I | I | I |
| Population, no | | | | | | | | | |
| OP | 174 | 170 | 128 | 103 | 77 | 48 | 39 | 89 | 89 |
| LAP | 179 | 170 | 253 | 101 | 76 | 51 | 34 | 82 | 82 |
| Tumour stage | | | | | | | | | |
| I | NA | NA | NA | 15% (OP)<br>11% (LAP) | 15% (OP)<br>17% (LAP) | NA | NA | NA | NA |
| II | NA | NA | NA | 38% (OP)<br>35% (LAP) | 38% (OP)<br>38% (LAP) | NA | NA | NA | NA |
| III | NA | NA | NA | 43% (OP)<br>45% (LAP) | 26% (OP)<br>36% (LAP) | NA | NA | NA | NA |
| IV | NA | NA | NA | 5% (OP)<br>10% (LAP) | 21% (OP)<br>9% (LAP) | NA | NA | NA | NA |
| Postoperative chemotherapy | NA | Recommended for 4 mo | 29% (OP)<br>28% (LAP) | Stage III or IV disease | 33% (OP)<br>14% (LAP) | NA | NA | NA | NA |
| Surgery | | | | | | | | | |
| Tumour distance from AV, cm | NA | 5.3 (OP)<br>5.6 (LAP) | NA | 6.2 (OP)<br>5.5 (LAP) | 12–15 cm | ≥ 5 cm | 8 (OP)<br>6 (LAP) | 8.6 (OP)<br>9.1 (LAP) | NA |
| Conversion rate | < 1% | 1% | 34% | 8% | 30% | 10% | 3% | 7% | NA |
| Surgeon experience | Experienced surgeon | 28–150 LAP | ≥ 20 LAP | Experienced team | Experienced surgeon | Experienced surgeon | Experienced surgeon | Experienced team | Experienced surgeon |

AV = anal verge; CLASICC = Conventional Versus Laparoscopic-Assisted Surgery in Patients with Colorectal Cancer; COREAN = Comparison of Open versus laparoscopic surgery for mid and low Rectal cancer After Neoadjuvant chemoradiotherapy; DFS = disease-free survival; LAP = laparoscopy; LR = local recurrence; NA = not available; OP = open surgery; OS = overall survival.

*This trial included patients with colon and rectum cancers. When available, data specific to rectal cancer are presented.

†As evaluated according to the American Society of Clinical Oncology and European Society for Medical Oncology gradation system (Table 1).

In 1992, M.Gagner reported the first laparoscopic liver resection under laparoscopy, which is also considered advanced surgery. (24).

The number of laparoscopic liver resections has increased exponentially worldwide since this first publication, notably in carcinological surgery (liver metastases of colorectal origin, hepatocellular carcinoma) (26) (Fig.54).

In his review Nguyen had surveyed all laparoscopic liver resections across 127 publications that included 2804 patients, and concluded that laparoscopy was associated with less morbidity, less pain, faster recovery, shorter hospital stay than open procedures, without compromising oncological clearance (26).

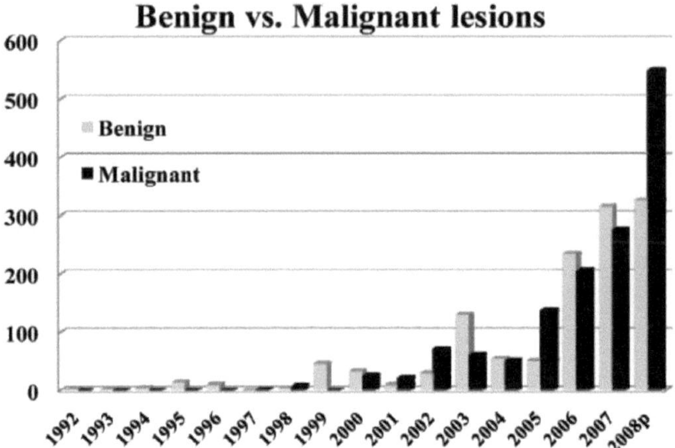


**Figure 54** Laparoscopic liver resections for benign and malignant pathologies reported in the literature (26).

Two consensus conferences on laparoscopic liver surgery have been held, the first in Louisville, USA, in 2008, the second in Morioka, Japan, in 2014. These conferences reviewed the current state of laparoscopic liver surgery, clarifying its indications and prospects, based on updated data from the literature and on questions put to the panels of world experts present at the two conferences.
More recently in 2017, Abu Hilal published the European guidelines (Southampton guidelines) for laparoscopic liver surgery (115).

In 2018 the results of the first randomized trial comparing laparoscopic versus conventional surgery in liver resections for metastases of colorectal origin were published (OSLO-COMET trial) (116). This Norwegian trial included 280 patients, 133 in the laparoscopic arm and 147 in the laparotomy arm. Postoperative complications and length of stay were lower in the laparoscopic arm, as was cost. The rate of healthy resection margins was equivalent in both arms.
These findings supported the implementation of laparoscopic liver surgery.

In our work, we wanted to improve the approach to patients presenting with CCMHS compared with the traditional approach, which is so debilitating that a minimally invasive laparoscopic approach to at least one of the two tumour sites seemed advantageous to patients in the light of the literature presented above, since laparoscopy had been validated for colorectal surgery and had become a standard for minor liver resections, why not combine the two in patients who, precisely because of the bifocal location of their tumors, had a problem with the approach?

The first cases of simultaneous laparoscopic resection of a colorectal tumor and its liver metastasis were reported in 2006.
T.M Geiger (28) reported a hepatic resection (coelio-assisted left lobectomy (hand-assisted)) followed by a laparoscopic sigmoid resection, with a simple postoperative course and good carcinological quality of the resection (Fig.55, Fig.56).

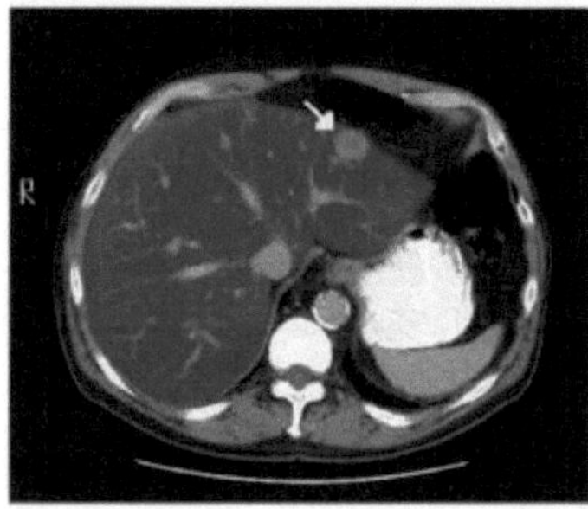


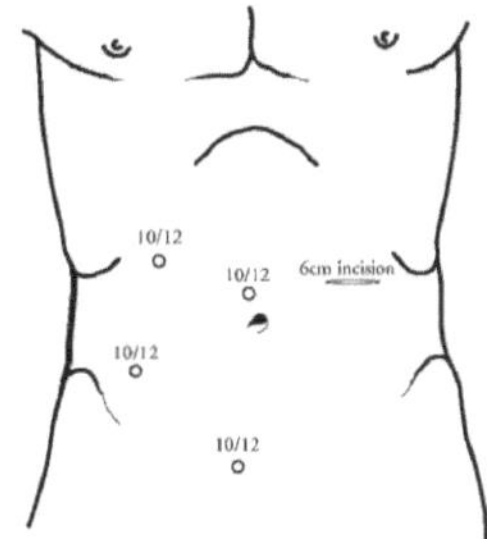


**Figure 55** Left lobe metastasis (28).

**Figure 56** Combined approach (28).

Also in 2006, K.L Leung (29) in the same journal, published another case report, this time of a totally laparoscopic resection combining an anterior resection for cancer of the upper rectum, followed by a left lobectomy for a double metastatic localization, in a 53-year-old patient, with a simple postoperative course and R0 quality resection of both tumour sites (Fig.57).

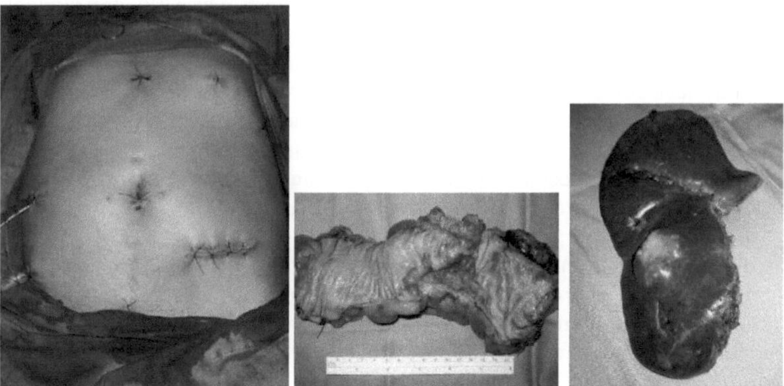

**Figure 57** Totally laparoscopic approach for anterior resection combined with left lobectomy (29).

Three types of approach have been described in the literature to date:

- The hybrid approach, which combines the laparoscopic and conventional approaches to two distinct tumour sites (18). The ″ hand assisted ″ laparoscopic surgery HALS , was also described by the authors in this approach (145).

- All laparoscopic: primary tumor and liver metastasis are removed laparoscopically (146)The use of the robot in this approach has also been described (147).

- Laparoscopic ″down staging″ surgery: with or without portal ligation, as part of two-stage hepatectomy, for patients with multiple bilobar metastases. The advantages of this approach have been described by P.Pessaux (39) who reported on the advantages of performing the first stage laparoscopically, thus benefiting from the classic advantages of laparoscopy in terms of rehabilitation, but also from a purely surgical point of view: the second stage is facilitated by the absence or reduction of adhesions associated with the first operation.

In the literature, the results of this new approach have been assessed on two fronts: firstly, technical feasibility, with morbidity and mortality assessment and conversion rate as the main objectives.
Secondly, a carcinological feasibility component, in which evaluation of the quality of resection (resection margins), the recurrence rate and the survival rate were the main objectives.

Since the first case report publications in 2006, the literature has been considerably enriched by other types of publication (monocentric series (Hatwell), etc.). (30)multicenter series (Ferretti) (35)systematic reviews (Lupinacci, Garritano) (34,37)), but no randomized study has yet been published to compare this new approach with the classic laparotomy approach, which is understandable since such randomization would raise ethical issues. However, the authors have compared their series with concomitant or historical series (conventional surgery), but they have also compared their series with concomitant series of patients who have undergone laparoscopic colorectal resection alone, as did Bretagnol (18) and Van der Poel (38). The aim of their comparison was to assess the effect of adding a liver stage to laparoscopic colorectal resection on morbidity and mortality. Their studies found no difference between the two groups.

In our work, we compared our experimental group (combined laparoscopic surgery) with the laparoscopic colorectal surgery group alone. Both groups were included during the same period, with patients operated on by the same surgeon and for a neoplastic pathology (to reduce bias).

In our study, all three types of approach described in the literature were performed, however ″ hand-assisted ″ laparoscopic surgery HALS was not used, nor was robotic surgery.
The number of patients in each approach was not equivalent.

Hybrid surgery made up the majority of our series, but laparoscopic colorectal surgery combined with laparoscopic liver surgery (liver resection, portal ligation or both) was performed in only 10 patients (25%).
To explain this high rate of hybrid surgery, we must refer to the location of liver metastases in our series, since in 65% of cases they were located in the posterior segments and often required complete mobilization of the right liver.
Laparoscopic approach to posterior segments is difficult (148) especially in the context of simultaneous surgery. To this end, difficulty scores for laparoscopic liver surgery have been reported by several authors and summarized in Ruben Ciria's publication (118) where 7 of the 11 scores presented considered tumour location as a factor of difficulty.
The purely laparoscopic approach for resection of liver metastases in our series had involved liver metastases localized in segments II and III, and only once in segment IVa but on a subcapsular lesion.

## E. Colorectal resection :

In our series, the primary tumor was colonic in 60% of cases and rectal in 40%. It was found in the right colon in 10% of cases, the sigmoid in 40% and the rest of the left colon in 10%.
Laparoscopic colorectal resection surgery was performed in the standard manner described in the methods section, with a few special features and findings in the context of this simultaneous surgery.

Twelve patients, i.e. 30% of our series, had a history of abdominal surgery. After statistical analysis of the results, only a history of midline incision was statistically associated with the occurrence of a severe incident, grade 2 according to the Oslo classification ($p = 0.013$), whereas a history of abdominal surgery was not a risk factor for intraoperative incident ($p = 0.095$) or conversion ($p = 0.704$). This can be explained by the importance of postoperative adhesions caused by the first operation in the case of a prior midline incision, which required us to perform extensive adhesiolysis each time (see video 2). Four patients had been approached via this type of incision, two for an occlusive syndrome in whom a near upstream colostomy had been performed, one patient had been operated on for a bulbar ulcer and the fourth had been operated on via an xypho-pubic route for the removal of a textiloma left over from a previous left nephrectomy.

Four patients had developed an occlusive syndrome during chemotherapy, all of whom underwent emergency surgery (three in other hospitals). A near upstream colostomy (sigmoid tumor) was performed in each case (twice by median approach and twice by elective approach).
During our laparoscopic approach, we noted that after the adhesiolysis period, the stoma itself allowed exposure of the left mesocolon and facilitated access to the mesenteric vessels (see video 2).

On the other hand, in all cases we had to take the stoma with us to the resection site, thereby increasing colonic sacrifice, which meant that we systematically had to unhook the left colonic angle to perform a tension-free colorectal anastomosis in these cases.

Four patients had a primary right colonic tumor, all had hepatic metastases on posterior segments. A hybrid approach was planned for each case.
For three patients, the colonic stage was performed laparoscopically (vascular ligations, colonic mobilization) with extracorporeal anastomosis via a right transverse incision. For the liver procedure, we had to add a midline incision to mobilize the liver and expose the metastases (segment VII).
In the fourth patient, conversion was decided upon due to intolerance of pneumoperitoneum, using a low Makuuchi incision which enabled us to complete the laparoscopic colonic resection and resection of posterior liver metastases.
The hybrid approach, as used for the first three patients, seems less interesting than for left-sided localizations.
Laparoscopic right colonic resection with intracorporeal anastomosis should be preferred, and patients with anteroinferior liver metastases should be selected. Or opt for totally laparoscopic surgery regardless of the location of the metastases.

Ten patients had received neoadjuvant radiotherapy, including 8 with short course radiotherapy, of whom 5 underwent immediate surgery.
During proctectomy in these patients, we noted the extent of edema during dissection of the mesorectum. This edema itself dissected the space between the fascia recti and the presacral fascia, which facilitated resection, but strict adherence to the correct plane was necessary, as any deviation from this plane exposed a risk of haemorrhage given the local inflammatory state (see video 1).
In one patient, edema extended into the mesocolon around the origin of the inferior mesenteric artery.

In two patients with a left primary tumour location (sigmoid, upper rectum), the resection procedure was widened to the right, combined with a Deloyer-type lowering manoeuvre and colorectal anastomosis. After the laparoscopic resection on the left, the complementary colonic resection was performed through the incision used for liver surgery.
This additional procedure was necessary after a lesion of Riolan's arch in one patient, while in the second patient it was necessary because the stoma created during the anterior occlusive syndrome was located in the transverse colon.
Even in the event of an incident or surgical surprise, conversion remains a solution of last resort in the surgeon's mind.
In the case of hybrid surgery, the incision used for the extraction of the surgical specimen is also used to prepare the colonic transplant for anastomosis (placement of the anvil), either as a median supraumbilical, subcutaneous or Makuuchi incision.
In order to facilitate preparation of the colonic transplant, we systematically mobilized the left colonic angle for all left colonic and rectal tumors.

The route of extraction of the colorectal resection specimen was the route used for liver surgery, in the case of hybrid surgery, or a Pfannenstiel incision, in the case of totally laparoscopic surgery or down staging with portal ligation.
There are a few exceptions:
In the case of abdominoperineal amputation, the part is removed perineally after turning.
One patient underwent trans-anal extraction for a tumor of the lower rectum.
In one patient, extraction was performed through the stomal orifice (see video 2) (Fig.58).

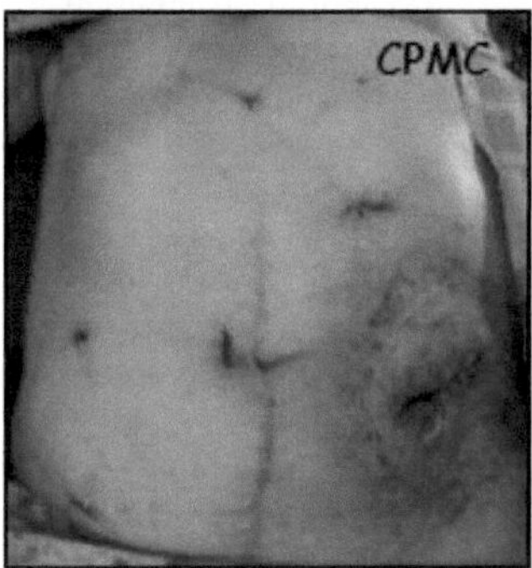


**Figure 58** Stomal orifice extraction. History of near proximal median colostomy (CPMC).

Drainage of the colorectal excision site was not systematically performed in 21 patients, mainly after rectal surgery.

## F. Liver surgery:

The hepatic time of combined surgery in our series consisted of either a minor hepatic resection of less than 3 segments (defined from the Brisbane 2000 terminology of hepatic anatomy and resections) (105)or portal ligation, or both.
Ten cases (25%) had undergone laparoscopic liver surgery.

### 1. Laparoscopic liver surgery:

The laparoscopic approach to the liver involved the addition of at least one 5 mm trocar at epigastric level, in addition to the trocars already used during the colorectal phase.
In the case of laparoscopic liver resection, we always started with the colorectal resection, followed by the liver resection, then finished by performing the anastomosis if we had to re-establish continuity.
We adopted this strategy to avoid the need for an additional incision in the event that laparoscopic liver resection could not be completed, since in this scenario, if

the colorectal resection specimen were extracted through a Pfannenstiel incision, the liver resection would have been performed through a subcutaneous or median incision, leaving the patient with 2 separate incisions at the end of the procedure. In all cases, our strategy enabled a single incision to be made.

In the literature, some authors started with the liver time, arguing that this was the most hemorrhagic time, and that in the event of major bleeding they could make do with the liver time, switching to a reverse strategy, since the prognosis is linked to the control of metastatic disease, even in the absence of bleeding, since liver surgery is performed at low PVC and on a ″versant sec″, a deleterious effect on a digestive anastomosis was feared, in addition to the effects of possible pedicle clamping.
Other authors systematically began with the colorectal stage, arguing that from a carcinological point of view, it was imperative to ensure R0 carcinological excision of the primary tumor before considering resection of liver metastases.

Laparoscopic liver resection procedures included wedges on segment III on three occasions, metastasectomies on segment III on two occasions, a metastasectomy on segment II in one patient, and a double metastasectomy III and IVa in another patient.

Laparoscopic portal ligation had been performed in six patients, 5 times on the right and once on the left.
It was performed 5 times after colorectal time, and once before colorectal time.

The peritoneum of the hepatic pedicle was then incised (posterior right in the case of right portal ligation, or anterior left in the case of left portal ligation), and the hepatic artery (right or left branch) was placed on lakes for better exposure. Next, the most posterior element of the hepatic pedicle, the portal vein, was dissected. A dissector was then passed around the portal branch to be ligated, using a wire to ensure that the contralateral branch had been ligated beforehand. A wire ligation was performed to reduce the diameter of the vein, enabling us to place at least one locked clip on the portal branch. We did not inject pure alcohol into the vein after ligation, as described in some publications.

Remaining liver volume gain averaged 59.48%, and differed from patient to patient. On follow-up scans, we observed reopacification by shunts of the territories affected by the ligation, to varying degrees and at different times. In the patient who had undergone ALPPS, a portal cavernoma had formed. Nevertheless, there was no ″ drop out ″ of patients, and all six patients had been reoperated, and in each case a major hepatectomy had been performed. In other words, the therapeutic strategy outlined at the outset was carried through to completion, enabling carcinological resection of the primary tumor and liver metastases.

## 2. **Laparotomy liver surgery:**

Laparotomy liver surgery was performed in association with laparoscopic removal of the colorectal tumor.

As previously mentioned, the approaches were either a median supraumbilical incision, a right subcostal incision or a Makuuchi incision.
The type of incision depended on the location of liver metastases (right liver/left liver) and whether or not complete mobilization of the right liver was required.
In our series, in 65% of cases they were located in the posterior segments, hence the frequent mobilization of the right liver and consequently the more frequent approach via a Makuuchi incision.
Hepatic clamping was prepared but not systematically, and we clamped 12 patients. Hepatic resection procedures ranged from simple metastasectomy, through non-anatomical wedge resections, to anatomical resections such as segmentectomy or bisegmentectomy (posterior sectoriectomy).
These resections could be combined in the same patient, but in total, less than three segments were resected each time, in line with the need to combine colorectal surgery with a minor resection.

Intraoperative ultrasound was used in 7 patients, for several purposes: firstly, to localize metastases already identified on preoperative CT/MRI scans, especially in the case of deep-seated metastases. It was also intended to clarify the vascular relationships of certain metastases to guide the surgical procedure, and in some cases of multiple metastases, to detect lesions not described on CT/MRI.
In our practice, ultrasound was effective for the first two purposes, but did not uncover any new lesions other than those described on CT or MRI.

Drainage of the hepatic resection site was not systematic, and a drain was left in 8 cases.

## G. Major hepatectomies / Portal ligation :

Six patients with bilobar liver metastases were candidates for two-stage hepatectomy.
The second major hepatic stage followed a first stage of colorectal resection and portal ligation, with or without clearance of a hemi-loan.
The second operation was carried out on average 16 weeks after the first operation, a longer time than described in the literature (8 ± 3 weeks). This could be explained by the patient's course after the first operation, who, after the convalescence period, begins interval chemotherapy, This is followed by a CT scan to assess the degree of hypertrophy and the status of metastatic disease, and then scheduling for surgery (after a second pre-anaesthetic assessment), which must be delayed until after the last course of chemotherapy, particularly if an antiangiogenic agent was added to the chemotherapy.

A total of four right hepatectomies had been performed, including one after ALPPS.
Left hepatectomy extended to the right anterior sector.
A posterior sectoriectomy extended to segment VIII.

These operations were performed by laparotomy, and the adhesions associated with the first operation were not numerous, and did not interfere with the second operation.

Two of the six patients experienced severe morbidity, necessitating revision surgery. Postoperative outcome was favorable.
Both patients had presented with liver recurrence; the first had been reoperated and resected, and was alive without recurrence at 25 months.
The second had presented an unresectable recurrence, and had been treated with medication. He was alive at 26 months.

These patients with synchronous bilobar liver metastases are unresectable from the outset, and cannot be treated by a single surgical procedure. To achieve complete resection of the neoplasia, a multi-stage oncosurgical approach is required. During this course, there is a real risk of progression of the metastatic disease, synonymous with the patient's exit from the therapeutic project or ″drop out ″ estimated in the literature at around one in five patients. In a single-center retrospective series of over 300 cases, Yamashita (149) reported that approximately 20% of patients who underwent portal embolization were not ultimately resected, mainly due to disease progression.
In some cases, it may also be due to insufficient liver hypertrophy despite embolization or portal ligation.

Comparing the efficacy of portal ligation versus portal embolization in the induction of hepatic hypertrophy has been the subject of several publications with discordant results, while some report the superiority of portal embolization (150 - 152) explaining its greater efficacy by the fact that it obstructs vessels, unlike portal ligation where shunts can revascularize territories initially excluded.
Other publications find no difference between the two techniques (153)both techniques may be ineffective because of the formation of a portal cavernoma.
In the era of evidence-based medicine, to draw conclusions we must refer to more powerful studies, in this sense, a metanalysis published in 2017 by C.J. Isfordink (154) in surgical oncology, had identified 21 studies eligible for analysis in the literature that included 1953 portal embolisations and 123 portal ligations, there was no significant difference in the rate of remaining future liver hypertrophy between the two techniques (PVE 43.2%, PVL 38.5%, $p = 0.39$). The number of liver resections cancelled for insufficient hypertrophy was significantly lower after portal ligation ($p = 0.002$). There was no postoperative difference in mortality or morbidity.

We chose portal ligation for several reasons:
-Firstly, because we were in a synchronous situation, with the primary tumor in place, which implied a first stage colorectal surgery.
This surgical time would allow abdominal exploration in search of a possible contraindication to resection, which would render the entire liver strategy obsolete.

-Secondly: because we had opted for minimally invasive laparoscopic surgery for this first stage, which would allow resection of the primary tumor and portal ligation in the same operation.
-Thirdly, because, although portal embolization is a minimally invasive procedure, it is not without morbidity. Several complications have been described in the literature (155)These include hemorrhage, hematoma, hemobilia, undesirable extension of embolization to territories that were not intended to be embolized (portal trunk by retrograde embolization, IV segment vein), venous thrombosis, infectious complications, etc.
Ultimately, our strategy enabled complete resection of the liver metastases.

In reviewing the literature, reported gains in future remaining liver volume (FFR) were variable, Robles (150) observed after portal ligation a median gain of 30% (21% - 60%), these findings were made after a median delay of 35 days (28d - 60d), in Isfordink's metanalysis (154) the mean rate of hypertrophy after portal embolization was 43.2%, and 38.5% after portal ligation; the interval between embolization or portal ligation and re-evaluation of volumetry varied between studies (2 to 8 weeks). Other results (156) concerning portal embolization are presented in Table 90 :

**Table 90** Left liver hypertrophy after right portal embolization (156).

**Tableau** . Hypertrophie du foie gauche après embolisation portale droite.

| *Références* | *Foie non tumoral* | *Matériel* | *Délai* | *Hypertrophie* |
|---|---|---|---|---|
| Goto et al. | Normal | Colle biologique | 2 semaines | 32 % |
| Imamura et al. | Normal et anormal | Colle biologique | 2 semaines | 31 % |
| Tanaka et al. | Fibrose F1 à F4 | Colle biologique | 2 semaines | 37 % |
| Harada et al. | – | Colle biologique | 3 semaines | 44 % |
| Elias et al. | Normal | Colle acrylique | 4 semaines | 70 % |
| Shimamura et al. | Fibrose F1 à F4 | Alcool | 2 semaines | 93 % |
| | | | 4 semaines | 111 % |

In our series, 5 patients had significant hypertrophy of the remaining future liver, and the mean gain in volume of the remaining future liver was 59.48%, higher than the rates reported by Isfordink. This could be explained by the longer time to surgery in our series, which averaged 15.8 weeks.

The temporal behavior of the non-embolized liver was studied (Fig.59) (155)it was reported that the regeneration rate increased during the first 3 weeks, followed by a plateau phase with a further slight increase in volume (157).

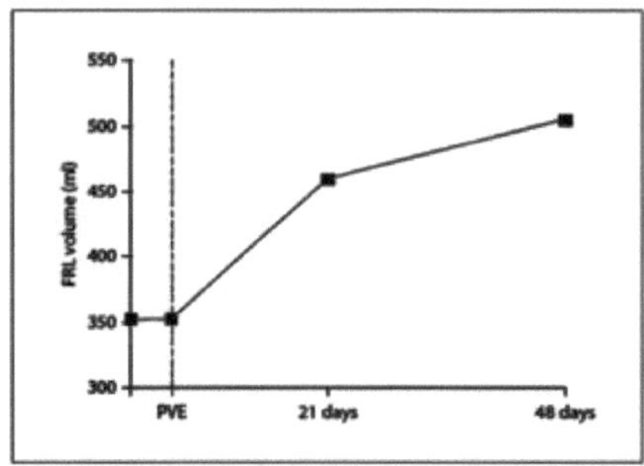


**Figure 59** Hypertrophy of the future remaining liver as a function of time (155).

Corrêa's publication (158) looked at the fate of the liver over a one-year period after right portal embolization in ten patients who had not been resected for various reasons.

During this year, the left liver had grown by a total of 83.4%. Of the total growth, 50% occurred 90 days after embolization and 75% after 230 days. These data confirm that atrophy on the treated side and compensatory hypertrophy on the contralateral side occur continuously until at least 360 days after embolization (Fig.60).

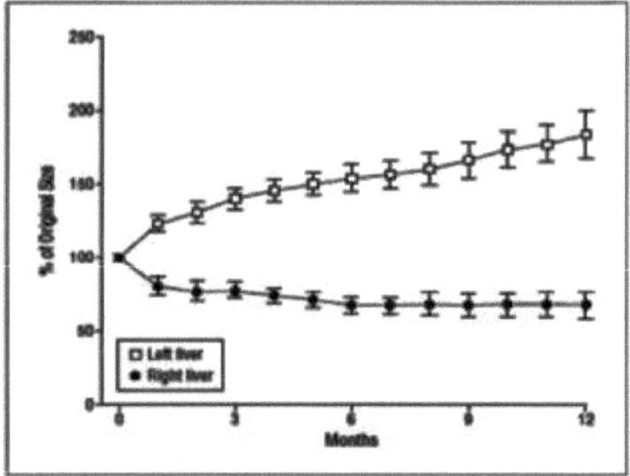


**Figure 60** Right liver atrophy and left liver hypertrophy in the Corrêa series. (158).

In our series, therefore, extending the time to surgery had a positive effect on the rate of hypertrophy, but at the same time there was a risk of disease progression.

The failure of portal ligation on hypertrophy was noted in one patient, and a purely anatomical cause was identified in him by analyzing the imaging. In fact, a portal anatomical variation of the type of stepped distribution of the portal vein existed in this patient.

The right portal vein, which had been clipped, supplied only the posterior area (Fig.61, Fig.62).

Systematic review of preoperative imaging is recommended for a better indication of the portal ligation procedure.

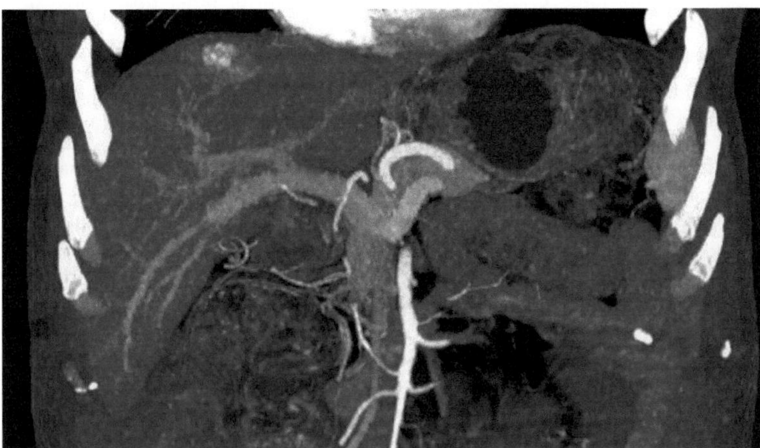

**Figure 61** Portal anatomical variation explaining failure of portal ligation in patient #3 (CPMC).

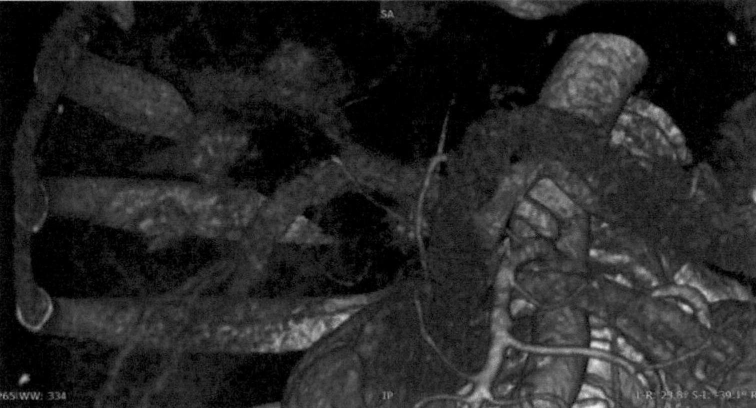


**Figure 62** 3D reconstruction of the same patient (CPMC).

These patients receive chemotherapy for long periods and undergo major liver resections, making them vulnerable to severe post-operative complications.

Carcinologically, these patients are also at high risk of recurrence.

Tumor biology plays an important role in this context.

That said, the goal remains to achieve R0 resection, the only guarantee of improved survival.

## H. Operating time :

The average operative time for our series was 323 min for total operative time, 221.8 min for colorectal time and 101.2 min for liver time.
Operating time for hybrid surgery was longer than for other procedures ($p$ = 0.017).
The duration of down-staging surgery was the shortest of the different procedures ($p$ = 0.041).
Conversion did not affect operating time ($p$ = 0.069).

In the literature, simultaneous laparoscopic surgery was chosen if the total duration of the preoperative procedure was < 8 hours (30).
This empirically fixed duration was considered a threshold that should not be exceeded, since the advantages of the laparoscopic approach would be lost and, what's more, additional morbidity could be observed.
In our series, the longest operation lasted 7 hours.

The median operative time for the simultaneous laparoscopic approach reported in Moris' systematic review (159) was 335.5 min (240 min - 495 min).

In our comparative study, between the experimental arm (simultaneous surgery) and the control arm (laparoscopic colorectal surgery), operative time was longer in the simultaneous surgery arm, with a highly significant difference ($p$ = 0.000). Liver time had a significant impact on total operative time.

In studies comparing simultaneous laparoscopic and laparotomy surgery, the laparoscopic approach prolonged operating time in some of the publications (33, 146,160).
Operative times were equivalent in others (36,,161,162).
On the other hand, Hu (163) reported a shorter operative time in the laparoscopic arm.
In our study, operative time was not a risk factor for morbidity ($p$ = 0.381).

## I. Postoperative rehabilitation:

Patients were systematically included in the enhanced rehabilitation protocol introduced in the department since 2017 for patients with colorectal cancer (AGER protocol).
The multimodal management of postoperative pain, which was an integral part of the protocol, combined with the laparoscopic approach, resulted in satisfactory postoperative pain control.
At 24$^{ème}$ hours and on a visual analog scale, 62.5% of patients had pain estimated at < 3/10.

Eating was resumed early, and an herbal tea was allowed on the evening of the operation.

Transit resumption was early, with 87.5% of patients resuming transit within the first 48 hours. Only one patient resumed transit up to postoperative day 4[ème] .

Ratti (146) also reported in his comparative study an earlier resumption of transit in the laparoscopic arm [3d (2-6) vs. 5d (2-7)] $p$ = 0.04.
The same findings were made in Gorgun's study (161) (2.9d ± 0.3 vs. 4.5d ± 0.3) $p$ = 0.003. Resumption of normal feeding was also earlier in the laparoscopic arm (4d ± 0.5 vs. 6.4d ± 0.5) $p$ = 0.001.

## J. Postoperative stay:

Postoperative hospital stay averaged 5.1 ± 2.58 days, with a median of 4 days and extremes of 3 and 17 days.
There was no significant difference in post-operative length of stay between the different types of surgical procedure (all laparoscopic, hybrid or down-staging surgery). There was also no difference in case of conversion.

In our comparative study (control arm vs. experimental arm), there was no significant difference in postoperative length of stay between the two arms (5.48 ± 2.81 days vs. 5.10 ± 2.58 days) $p$ = 0.537.

Eight patients underwent post-operative care in the intensive care unit, with an average stay of 3.75 days and a median of 2.5 days, with extremes ranging from 1 to 13 days.

In our series, length of postoperative stay was statistically linked in univariate analysis with overall morbidity ($p$ = 0.030), mild morbidity *($p$ = 0.006)* and severe morbidity ($p$ = 0.002).

ICU stay was statistically associated with severe morbidity ($p$ = 0.036).

In our comparative study, multivariate analysis of morbidity-related variables for all patients in both arms (80 patients) identified length of postoperative stay ($p$ = 0.006), female gender *($p$ = 0.016)* and age ≥ 65 years ($p$ = 0.045).

One of the advantages of laparoscopy over laparotomy is the shortening of the postoperative stay; this has been verified by several comparative studies between the simultaneous laparoscopic and conventional approach (33,146,161,163 - 166).

## K. Associated treatments :

### 1. Radiotherapy:

In metastatic situations, there is no standard for the management of rectal cancer (167).

In this situation, we opted for the short protocol (8/10 patients), with immediate surgery in 5 patients.
The short 5×5 grays protocol with immediate surgery meets the two requirements of this situation, the introduction of neoadjuvant treatment for a T3 and or N+ rectal tumor, without lengthening the time to management of metastatic disease.

In two patients, CAP 50 RCC had been administered: the first patient had a T3 strong tumor of the lower rectum associated with a single synchronous liver metastasis, the second patient had a T3 strong tumor of the middle rectum associated with a single synchronous liver metastasis.
Post-radiotherapy re-evaluation revealed a reduction in rectal tumour volume in both cases. However, in the case of liver metastases, one patient remained stable, while the other showed significant volumetric progression.
Progression of metastatic disease after RCC is a real risk, since the protocol itself lasts 5 weeks and surgery is performed after 6-8 weeks.
In our practice, it would be advisable to discuss a reverse strategy when a long protocol (RCC) is required.

## 2. Chemotherapy / Targeted therapy :

Chemotherapy alone or combined with targeted therapy had been administered preoperatively to control metastatic disease in 29 patients, or 72.5% of cases.
In 11 patients (27.5%), surgery was performed either immediately or after radiotherapy. Of these, 10 patients had metastatic disease of limited extent (one or two small nodules) that was resectable from the outset, and chemotherapy was not chosen at the start of treatment because of the risk of disappearance of liver lesions. The eleventh patient presented with a stenosing sigmoid tumour that was beginning to become symptomatic, and was associated with two small liver metastases. Also in this patient, chemotherapy had not been chosen at the start of treatment, given the ″symptomatic ″ nature of the primary tumour and the easy resectability of the liver metastases.

In the other patients, the protocol depended on whether the liver metastases were resectable or potentially resectable at the time of initial radiological evaluation.
Perioperative chemotherapy FOLFOX 4 or CAPOX in the case of resectable metastases was used in 11 patients.
Neoadjuvant chemotherapy, combining FOLFOX or CAPOX chemotherapy with targeted therapy (such as antiangiogenic or anti-EGFR antibodies, depending on RAS status) in 18 patients.

Perioperative chemotherapy indicated for resectable metastases (grade C recommendation) (52)has been introduced since the work of Nordlinger (92) who found a gain in progression-free survival in the perioperative chemotherapy arm. The long-distance results of this study were published in 2013 (93)There was no difference in 5-year overall survival between the two arms.

In the case of potentially resectable metastases (52)it is recommended to use a CT protocol with a high response rate (objective responses according to RECIST1.1) with a view to secondary resectability: (tri-CT or bi-CT) plus biotherapy (94).
In our series, tri-CT had not been administered.
The average number of preoperative courses for all types of chemotherapy was 5.97, with a median of 6 and extremes of 3 to 13 courses.
In the case of perioperative chemotherapy, the average number of preoperative courses was 4.
In the case of neoadjuvant chemotherapy, the number of courses was higher in some patients, since the disease was re-evaluated every two months until a response allowing resection was achieved.
Of the 29 patients who had received chemotherapy ± targeted therapy preoperatively, 12 showed a partial response and 17 stable metastatic liver disease.
There was no progression with chemotherapy.
No complete responses were received.
On the basis of these results, we can say that tumor control by chemotherapy was good.

Data on chemotherapy toxicity were not complete, and many missing data prevented us from analyzing the results in this respect. Nevertheless, we noted a single case of severe chemotherapy toxicity, which obliged us to postpone surgery after a protocol of perioperative chemotherapy followed by short radiotherapy in a patient with adenocarcinoma of the middle rectum associated with a single liver metastasis. The toxicity was dual, grade 3 hematological and renal.

## L. Perioperative results:

### 1. Perioperative adverse events:

In 1992, Clavien et Coll (168) proposed a classification of postoperative complications, which has since been validated (125,126) . Postoperative complication was defined as "any initial deviation from the expected operative course", and included asymptomatic complications such as arrhythmia and atelectasis. In their publication, the authors of the classification had differentiated the complication of :

- *Failure* to cure": where surgery, although performed without complications, fails to achieve its objective. (For example, a residual tumor after surgery).
- Sequela: is a "side effect" of surgery that is inherent to the procedure (for example, the inability to walk after a leg amputation).

However, the limits of this classification have been noted in practice, as it refers to complications, ignores all inconsequential matters (e.g., an aortic wound with simple sequelae after conversion will appear nowhere in a Clavien evaluation), and does not claim to take into account the specificity of laparoscopy (e.g., conversion) and surgical hazards, which are nevertheless instructive to record and monitor.

Morbidity is also underestimated at discharge. In a study by club coelio (169) the rate of uncomplicated patients fell from 93% at discharge to 86.53% at one month. In addition, the recent development of outpatient surgery and improved rehabilitation after surgery requires a more detailed assessment of the patient's outcome after discharge.

Consideration of intraoperative incidents is becoming necessary, especially in the context of laparoscopic surgery; recently, Kazaryan et al. (123) have proposed the Oslo classification, specifying these intraoperative events on the basis of Satava's work on the evaluation of surgical errors (124).

Moreover, in the case of conversion, whether it is preemptive or reactive must be known, as postoperative morbidity is increased in the event of an intraoperative incident and in reactive conversions.
It seems certain that the notion of postoperative complications must give way to that of perioperative adverse events (Fig.63).

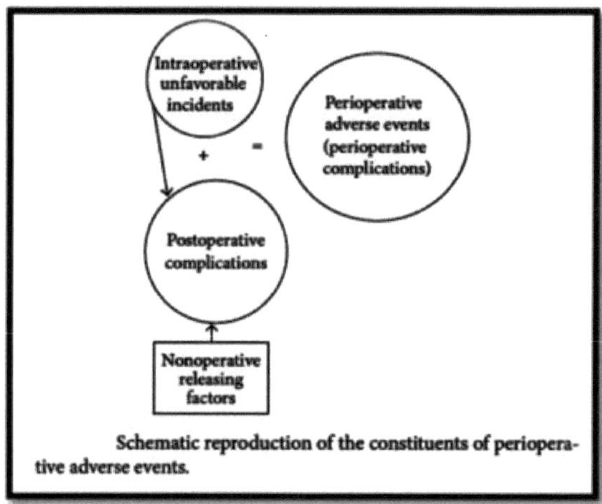


**Figure 63** Constituents of perioperative adverse events according to Kazaryan (123).

In 2013 K.Slankamenac (127)had proposed a new classification to complement the Clavien classification, the CCI (The Comprehensive Complication Index) described as a new continuous scale to measure surgical morbidity.

This is measured online by accessing www.assessurgery.com to use the CCI® calculator, a tool for assessing overall patient morbidity. The Comprehensive Complication Index (CCI®) is based on the Clavien-Dindo classification of complications, and takes into account every complication arising after an operation. Overall morbidity is reflected on a scale from 0 (no complications) to 100 (death) (appendix 8).

In 2017 Clavien (170)reviewed this new classification in a publication assessing its practical application. He concluded that the ICC added value to the Clavien-Dindo classification in patients with more than one complication, especially after major surgery. Its value increased with longer observation time after surgery (> 3 months).

## *a) Operating incidents :*

Intraoperative incidents in our series had been classified according to the Oslo classification, incorporating the character of the conversion (Table 91).

**Table 91** Oslo classification (169).

| | |
|---|---|
| Grade 0 | Aucun incident peropératoire |
| Grade I | Incident sans conséquence peropératoire |
| Grade II | Incident peropératoire avec conséquence traitée ou cours de l'intervention y compris transfusion sanguine et conversion |
| IIp | Conversion préemptive, avant l'incident ou accident |
| IIr | Conversion réactive, après l'incident ou accident |
| Grade III | Incident ou complication non reconnue au cours de l'intervention avec conséquence postopératoire |

In our series, intraoperative incidents of anaesthetic or surgical nature occurred in 10 patients, i.e. 25% of the total. They were grade 1 in 4 patients and grade 2 in 6.

We classified these incidents according to their impact on a change in surgical strategy. Grade 1 incidents were dealt with intraoperatively, without any change in the course of the operation, whereas grade 2 incidents required us to change our attitude (e.g. conversion, abandoning an operative time, widening a resection, transfusion, etc.).
The risk factor for the occurrence of intraoperative incidents in our series was the presence of comorbidities ($p$ = 0.049), while severe incidents were more closely linked to the existence of a history of abdominal surgery ($p$ = 0.037), and more specifically a history of a midline incision ($p$ = 0.013). In this situation, the importance of adhesions leads to a release time with risks of visceral or vascular wounds.
An intraoperative transfusion following a hemorrhagic accident (controlled without conversion) was also noted.

In the literature, few studies provide information on intraoperative incidents using the Oslo classification, which is relatively recent (123) (published in 2013), although the following are frequently cited: conversion and its cause, and transfusions.
Van der Poel's recent publication in 2019 of the results of a multicenter comparative study using a propensity score, between combined laparoscopic surgery and laparoscopic colorectal surgery alone (38)The Oslo classification was used to compare perioperative outcomes between the two groups (Table 92).

**Table 92** Incidents according to Oslo classification (38).

| | LLCR ($n=61$) | LCR ($n=61$) | $p$ |
|---|---|---|---|
| Operative time, min, median (IQR) | 206 (166–308) | 197 (148–231) | 0.057 |
| Blood loss, ml, median (IQR) | 200 (100–700) | 75 (5–200) | 0.011 |
| Conversion | 3 (5) | 5 (8) | 0.687 |
| Peroperative incidents, Oslo classification | | | 0.237 |
| None | 52 (85) | 56 (92) | |
| Grade 1 | 6 (10) | 4 (7) | |
| Grade 2 | 3 (5) | 1 (2) | |
| Grade 3 | 0 | 0 | |

In the combined laparoscopic surgery arm, he reported 10% Grade 1 incidents and 5% Grade 2 incidents.
No Grade 3 incidents were reported.

### *b) Conversion :*

In our series, the conversion rate was 7.5%.
Conversion was preemptive in one patient and reactive in two.
The causes of conversion were as follows:
- Adherent abdomen.
- Intolerance of pneumoperitoneum.
- The discovery of a T4 tumor infiltrating neighboring organs.

Statistical analysis in search of risk factors leading to conversion in our series highlighted the degree of severity of the intraoperative incident according to the grades of the Oslo classification ($p = 0.044$) and the degree of parietal infiltration on anatomopathological study ($p = 0.011$).

There was no significant difference in the conversion rate between our two study arms (7.5% CSIM vs. 10% CCRL) with a ($p = 0.500$).

The conversion rates reported in the main published studies evaluating the combined laparoscopic approach are summarized in (table 93) :

**Table 93** Conversion rates in the literature.

| Author | Type of study | Workforce | Conversion rates |
|---|---|---|---|
| Moris (159) | Systematic review | 199 | 0 - 10 % |
| Garritano (37) | Systematic review | 150 | 0,7 % |
| Lupinacci(34) | Systematic review | 39 | 0 % |
| Ferretti (35) | Multicentric | 142 | 4,9 % |
| Ratti (32) | Monocentric comparative | 69 | 0 % |
| Van der poel(38) | Multicentric comparative | 61 | 5 % |
| CPMC | Unicentric comparative | 40 | 7,5 % |

Our conversion rate was comparable to that reported in the literature.

## *c) Transfusion :*

Four patients had been transfused perioperatively, including three intraoperatively.

Postoperative transfusion was counted as Clavien grade II postoperative morbidity. It was decided on in the inpatient unit following a fall in hemoglobin level with bleeding externalized through the drain. The transfusion volume was two packed red blood cells.

Three patients underwent intraoperative transfusion, in one case following a bleeding incident.

In the other two cases, it was decided at the end of the procedure (which had gone without incident), in a cardiopathic patient with a preoperative hemoglobin level of 9.9 g/dl, and an ASA I patient with a preoperative hemoglobin level of 8.2 g/dl. The transfusion volume was a single packed red blood cell in the patient with the bleeding incident, and two packed red blood cells in the other two patients.

The perioperative transfusion rate was 10%.

Only a few publications have specified the transfusion rate in the results. In his multicenter series, Ferretti (35) reported a rate of 8.5%, transfusion was a risk factor for postoperative complications in his univariate analysis. In our study, intraoperative transfusion was not associated with the occurrence of a postoperative complication ($p=0.310$).

Blood loss is more frequently reported in the literature, and provides a basis for assessment and comparison.

At the start of our study, we had made some estimates of blood loss, but these did not seem reliable to us, as the method used for estimation was subject to frequent errors, which led us not to take these calculations into account when analyzing the results. Instead, we took into account transfusion, which can be a consequence of high blood loss. Transfusion volumes did not exceed two packed red blood cells per patient in our series (four patients transfused).

Simultaneous laparoscopic surgery results in less blood loss than the conventional approach. All the comparative studies (8 studies) cited in Moris' systematic review (159) reported less blood loss in the laparoscopic arm. The difference was significant in 4 studies (146,162,164,166).

## 2. **Postoperative morbidity and mortality:**

### *a) Postoperative morbidity and mortality at 30 days:*

In our series, there was no 30-day operative mortality. In the largest multicenter series of patients undergoing simultaneous laparoscopic surgery, Ferretti (35) reported a mortality rate of 2.1% (3 patients died out of 142 included), but it should be noted that 31.7% of patients in this series were classified as ASA III; in our series, they represented 5% of the total. The three deaths reported were due to either a surgical complication (hemorrhage) or a medical complication (acute coronary syndrome).
Lupinacci (34) reported zero mortality in his systematic review of simultaneous laparoscopic resection; he included 39 patients from 14 publications, retaining only liver resections ≥ 2 segments.
Francesca Ratti (32) reported a mortality rate of 1.4%, with one patient dying out of 69 included for hybrid surgery, presenting with severe liver failure. In her series, hepatic resection was major in 18.9% of cases and enlarged in 4.3%, which could explain the risk of postoperative liver failure.
In our series, simultaneous liver resection was always a minor resection. No cases of postoperative liver failure were observed.
Garritano (37) in his systematic review published after Lupinacci's, had included purely laparoscopic simultaneous resections excluding the hybrid route and the "Hand assisted". One hundred and fifty patients had been included, drawn from 20 publications. The mortality rate was 1.3% (2 patients died).
Another more recent systematic review published by D.Moris (159) included simultaneous purely laparoscopic resections. One hundred and ninety-nine patients were included, drawn from 12 publications. Of these, 139 patients were included in comparative studies. The reported mortality rate was 1%.
Other publications evaluating the simultaneous laparoscopic approach had reported a zero mortality rate (10,30,171 - 173).

To optimize results, it is essential to select patients for a simultaneous strategy. This strategy is aimed at patients in good general condition, with stabilized and controlled comorbidities if present, and the series published on the evaluation of laparoscopy in this situation are often series of selected patients.

Regarding postoperative morbidity, Ferretti (35) (international multicenter study on 142 patients) reported an overall morbidity of 31%, divided into specific morbidity 15.5% and general morbidity 15.5%. Of the specific morbidity, colorectal complications accounted for 7.7%, and hepatic complications for 7.7%.
The most frequent colorectal complication was anastomotic fistula (8/11).
The most frequent hepatic complication was biliary collection (6/11), followed by hemorrhage (3/11).
According to Clavien's classification, minor complications (I, II) accounted for 36.36% of the total, major complications (III,IV,V) 63.64% of the total.
This high proportion of major complications could be explained by the inclusion of patients in this study, 31.7% of whom were classified as ASA III.

In our series, the overall morbidity rate at 30 days was 27.5% (11/40). Of the 11 patients, 03 had colorectal complications (fistula, collection and disorders related to the protective ileostomy), 01 patient a hepatic complication.
According to the Clavien classification, minor complications (I, II) accounted for 81.82% and major complications (III) for 18.18%.
Minor complications predominated over major ones.
Compared with Ferretti's series, these results reflect a population with fewer comorbidities (ASA III = 5%) and less extensive liver resection.

In literature, Francesca Ratti's series (32) is closer to our own, since it included 69 patients operated on using a hybrid approach.
The overall morbidity rate was 24.6%, with three colorectal fistulas and 3 biliary fistulas reported.
Mild Clavian morbidity (I, II) accounted for the majority (82.35%) of complications, while major morbidity (III, IV,V) accounted for 17.65%.

Stefano Garritano (37) in his systematic review of the combined laparoscopic approach, included 150 patients from 20 published studies. The overall morbidity rate was 18%, with six patients having colorectal complications and 5 patients having hepatic complications. The minor liver resection rate was 89.3% (134/150).

Lupinacci (34) in a systematic review preceding that of Garritano, had included 39 patients from 14 publications. This small number for a systematic review is explained by one of the inclusion criteria in the study, since Lupinacci had only considered liver resections ≥ 2 segments. He reported morbidity in 6 patients, but this was difficult to analyze in some publications, as he included subgroups from certain series.

In his review D.Moris (159) reported an overall morbidity rate of 19.9%.

Furthermore, in studies comparing the new laparoscopic approach with the conventional approach (combined laparotomy surgery), the feasibility of the new approach was assessed by comparing immediate results (morbi-mortality, conversion rate, quality of excision) and, in some studies, distant oncological results (survival, recurrence).
The morbi-mortality of the two groups in the main comparative studies cited in D.Moris's systematic review is summarized in (table 94).

**Table 94** Short-term results of main comparative studies (159).

| Authors | Operative time, min (range) | Median ESTIMATE BLOOD LOSS, mL | Conversion rate, % | Flatus passing, d, (range) | Diet start, d, (range) | Complications | Hospital stay, d | 30-d mortality, % |
|---|---|---|---|---|---|---|---|---|
| Comparative studies (OSR vs LSR patients) | | | | | | | | |
| Chen et al[24] (2011) | 342 ± 38 vs 350 ± 45 P > 0.05 | 590 ± 85 vs 275 ± 96 P < 0.05 | 0 (0) | 2 vs 2 P < 0.05 | N/a | 9 vs 8 P > 0.05 | 16 ± 2.5 vs 12 ± 1.5 P < 0.05 | 0 vs 0 |
| Hu et al[25] (2012) | 350 ± 46 vs 313 ± 44 P < 0.05 | 273 ± 93 vs 258 ± 111 P > 0.05 | 0 (0) | N/a | N/a | 0 vs 1 | 11.2 ± 1.8 vs 8.5 ± 1.9 P < 0.05 | 0 vs 0 |
| Takasu et al[26] (2013) | 466 ± 107 vs 472 ± 90 P = 0.92 | 496 ± 191 vs 152 ± 128 P < 0.02 | 0 (0) | N/a | N/a | 2 vs 1 P > 0.05 | 36.1 ± 24.9 vs 16.2 ± 6.1 P = 0.08 | 0 vs 0 |
| Jung et al[27] (2014) | 244 (149-375) vs 290 (183-551) P = 0.008 | 250 vs 325 P = 0.35 | 0 (0) | 3 (2-8) vs 3 (1-4) P = 0.1 | 4.5 (2-16) vs 3 (1-11) P < 0.001 | 10 vs 4 P = 0.06 8 vs 1 DC ≤ II 2 vs 3 DC ≥ III | 10.5 (8-23) vs 8 (5-23) P = 0.001 | 0 vs 0 |
| Ratti et al[28] (2016) | 310(150-540) vs 420 (170-720) P = 0.03 | 600 (200-1300) vs 350 (100-1000) P = 0.02 | 1 (4) | 5 (2-7) vs 3 (2-6) P = 0.04 | 4 (3-9) vs 3 (2-8) P = 0.06 | 12 vs 6 p = 0.78 | 12 (7-35) vs 9 (4-17) p = 0.02 | 0 vs 0 |
| Ivanecz et al[29] (2017) | 257 ± 66.8 vs 261 ± 92.8 P = 0.91 | 170 (70-230) vs 105 (30-180) P = 0.23 | 0 (0) | N/a | N/a | 5 vs 3 P = 0.65 2 vs 2 DC ≤ II 3 vs 1 DC ≥ III | 11.5 (10-33) vs 8 (8-12) P = 0.044 | 0 vs 0 |
| Gorgun et al[30] (2017) | 341 ± 27 vs 321 ± 35 P = 0.85 | 578 ± 116 vs 347 ± 37 P = 0.70 | 0 (0) | 4.5 ± 0.3 vs 2.9 ± 0.3 P = 0.003 | 6.4 ± 0.5 vs 4 ± 0.5 P = 0.001 | 13 vs 1 P = 0.016 | 10 ± 0.9 vs 6.4 ± 0.8 P = 0.001 | 1 vs 0 |
| Xu et al[31] (2017) | 248.35 ± 79.97 vs 246.75 ± 78.20 P = 0.949 | 300 (162.5-575) vs 175 (100-275) P = 0.024 | 0 (0) | N/a | N/a | 5 vs 3 P = 0.693 | 12 (10-16.25) vs 9 (8.25-11.75) P = 0.029 | 0 vs 0 |

Abbreviations: DC, Dindo-Clavien classification of complications; ESTIMATE BLOOD LOSS, estimated blood loss; LSR, laparoscopic synchronous resection; N/a, not available; OSR, open synchronous resection.

The rate of postoperative complications was comparable between the two groups in the studies (33,162 - 166,174).

In Gorgun's study (161) there was a significant difference ($p$ = 0.016) in favor of the laparoscopy group.

Other comparative studies not cited in Moris' review, such as the (32,36, 160,175) found no difference in the rate of postoperative morbidity between the two groups.

As did Van Der Poel (38) and Bretagnol (18)we compared short-term results between two groups of patients. An experimental group undergoing combined laparoscopic surgery and a control group undergoing laparoscopic colorectal surgery alone. Both authors found no significant difference in postoperative morbidity between these two groups, $p$ = 0.69 for Bretagnol and $p$ = 0.481 for Van Der Poel . In our comparison, too, there was no difference between the two groups in overall morbidity ($p$ = 0.606), mild morbidity ($p$ = 1.000) and severe morbidity ($p$ = 0.338).
Analysis of morbidity risk factors for the entire population (in both arms) did not find that membership of either group influenced the occurrence of more complications. What did have an impact on overall morbidity in the total population of both study arms were female gender and age > 65.

**Table 95** Morbidity-mortality rates in the literature.

In the univariate analysis of factors associated with overall morbidity in the experimental arm, the following were identified:
Anemia (revealing symptom) ($p$ = 0.039), neoadjuvant treatment ($p$ = 0.039), preoperative chemotherapy ($p$ = 0.027), number of liver resections ($p$ = 0.035), occurrence of an intraoperative incident (Oslo) ($p$ = 0.045) and postoperative stay ($p$ = 0.030).
While the first 5 factors are considered risk factors, the post-op stay is more a consequence of morbidity.
In multivariate analysis, only anemia ($p$ = 0.046) and the number of liver resections ($p$ = 0.018) were independent factors in morbidity.

Concerning factors related to mild morbidity (Clavien I, II), univariate analysis had identified 5 factors:
Anemia (telltale symptom) ($p$ =0.016), neoadjuvant treatment ($p$ = 0.016), preoperative chemotherapy ($p$ = 0.007), clamping ($p$ = 0.025) and postoperative stay ($p$ = 0.006).

For factors associated with severe morbidity (Clavien III), univariate analysis identified 4 factors:
The number of preoperative chemotherapy courses ($p$ = 0.008), the occurrence of an intraoperative incident (Oslo) ($p$ = 0.010), postoperative stay ($p$ =0.002) and ICU stay ($p$ = 0.036).

Table 95 summarizes the morbidity and conversion rates of the main publications in the literature. The results of our series are also reported in the table.

| Study | Type | Workforce | Morbidity | Mortality | Conversion |
|---|---|---|---|---|---|
| Ferretti 2015 | Multi-centric | 142 | 31 % | 2,1 % | 4,9 % |
| Lupinacci 2014 | Systematic review | 39 | 15,4 % | 0 % | 0 % |
| Ratti 2015 | Unicentric | 69 | 24,6 % | 1,4 % | 0 % |
| Garritano 2016 | Systematic review | 150 | 18 % | 1,3 % | 0,7 % |
| Moris 2019 | Systematic review | 199 | 19,9 % | 1 % | 0 - 10 % |
| V.D poel 2019 | Multi-centric | 61 | 15 % | 0 % | 5 % |
| CPMC | Uni-centric | 40 | 27,5 % | 0 % | 7,5 % |

### b) *Morbidity and mortality at 90 days:*

As reported in the previous chapter, it has been observed that when the postoperative monitoring period was lengthened, the detection of new complications was frequent, in the Club Coelio study (169) the rate of uncomplicated patients fell from 93% at discharge to 86.53% at one month. It must therefore be recognized that accounting for a complication should not be limited to the hospitalization period or the 30-day post-operative period. The 90-day period is increasingly used in publications to report mortality or morbidity.
In our series, we did not record any mortality at 90 days, but one patient suffered additional morbidity classified as IIIa, in the form of a radiologically drained hepatectomy pocket collection.

## M. Anatomopathological study :

In assessing the feasibility of the technique, in addition to morbidity and mortality results and the conversion rate, the quality of excision is an oncological criterion that can be assessed immediately.
In our series, histological analysis of colorectal resection specimens revealed adenocarcinoma (well or moderately differentiated) in 90% of cases.
Mucinous adenocarcinoma was found in 3 cases (7.5%).
A complete histological response after perioperative chemotherapy had been observed in a colonic tumor.
On liver resection specimens, adenocarcinoma was also in the majority (80%), but the rate of complete histological response was higher, involving 6 patients (17.14%).
One patient after perioperative chemotherapy and 5 patients after neoadjuvant chemotherapy. The targeted therapy used in these 5 patients was an anti EGFR in 3 cases (Panitumumab 2 cases, Cetuximab 1 case) or an anti-angiogenic in 2 cases (Bevacizumab).
Concerning the quality of resection, on the primary tumor 95% of resections were R0. The circumferential margin was <1mm in two patients after proctectomy.
On resection of liver metastases, out of 56 specimens analyzed, 4 had a margin <1mm, i.e. R1.
This gives us an R0 resection rate of 92.8% based on the number of parts analyzed, and an R0 resection rate of 90% based on the number of patients.
Ferretti (35) in his multicenter study of 142 patients reported an R0 resection rate of liver metastases of 93%, Ratti (146) in his comparative study, reported 100% R0 liver resection in 25 patients and 96% R0 colorectal resection.
Hatwell (30) in his series of 51 patients (including 44 hybrid procedures) reported 100% R0 resection of the primary tumor and 82.35% R0 resection of liver metastases.
Gorgun (161) reported 85.7% R0 resection of liver metastases.
Ratti (32) in another study of 69 patients operated on using a hybrid procedure, reported an R0 colorectal resection rate of 97.1% and an R0 resection rate of

97.1% for liver metastases. Our R0 resection rates were within the ranges reported in the literature (table 96).

**Table 96** Surgical resection margins after simultaneous surgery.

| Study | Type | Workforce | Primary R0 | R0 Metas |
|---|---|---|---|---|
| Ferretti 2015 | Multi cent | 142 | - | 93 % |
| Hatwell 2013 | Uni cent | 51 | 100% | 82,35 % |
| Ratti 2016 | Uni cent | 25 | 96 % | 100 % |
| Gorgun 2017 | Uni cent | 14 | - | 85,7 % |
| Ratti 2015 | Uni cent | 69 | 97,1 % | 97,1 % |
| CPMC | Uni cent | 40 | 95 % | 92,8 % |

In addition, the quality of mesorectal excision was good in all laparoscopic patients after proctectomy.

Concerning curage, the mean number of nodes in the curage was 15.55 with a median of 12.5 and extremes ranging from 1 to 54 nodes.

This average is in line with the number of lymph nodes required by the TNM classification; nevertheless, despite a standardized surgical technique, we observed an insufficient number of lymph nodes in some patients.

By statistically analyzing patient subgroups, it was found that patients who had received chemotherapy preoperatively had significantly fewer nodes in the curage (13.31 vs. 21.45) ($p$ = 0.034) compared to patients who had not received chemotherapy preoperatively.

This notion has been reported in several publications; the effect of CCR on curage in rectal surgery had been evaluated in Amajoyi's study (176) who found a mean number of nodes of 9 with a median of 7 in proctectomy specimens after RCC, and a mean number of nodes of 13 with a median of 10 in proctectomy specimens from patients who had not received neoadjuvant treatment, the difference being significant ($p$ = 0.001). Chang (177) made the same findings regarding the reduction in the number of lymph nodes removed (6.68 ± 4.74 vs. 11.54 ± 6.44, $p < 0.010$), but introduced a new concept: the lymph node ratio remained stable between the two groups (0.122 ± 0.24 vs. 0.161 ± 0.23, $p = 0.361$).

Also Hiroshi Sawayama (178) reported the effects of preoperative chemotherapy on lymph node status, vascular invasion and primary tumor in metastatic patients. In our study, it was preoperative chemotherapy that had an impact on the number of lymph nodes in the curage and not radiotherapy.

The effect of preoperative chemotherapy on liver metastases was well known. In the case of primary tumors, the more frequent use of chemotherapy in a synchronous situation (primary in place) has led to the observation of therapeutic effects on colorectal tumors. Karoui (179) in a series of 38 metastatic patients (16 of whom had received chemotherapy preoperatively), observed a major histological response in 70% of colorectal cancers. The response of the primary tumor to chemotherapy and that of the corresponding hepatic metastasis were correlated.

In our series, we noted two RCRG1 therapeutic responses in colonic tumors after perioperative FOLFOX chemotherapy in one case and neoadjuvant CAPOX + cetuximab chemotherapy in the other.
There was no RCRG1 response in rectal tumors after radiotherapy, which could be explained by the fact that in our series of metastatic patients we favored a short protocol with immediate surgery. The fact of not deferring surgery does not allow radiotherapy to achieve down staging or downsizing.
Chemotherapy resulted in complete sterilization of liver metastases in 6 patients (20.69%), and a major response (TRG1 - TRG2) in 12 patients (41.38%), which is considered a good prognostic factor. (180).
The 8ème edition of the TNM classification was used, and there was a difference in patient distribution between the pre-therapeutic cTNM (clinical) and post-resection pTNM (pathological) classifications (table 97).
Several factors are responsible for this difference, including neoadjuvant treatment, which is responsible for down-staging in some patients (e.g. T0N0M1), and over- or under-assessment of the degree of parietal or lymph node infiltration on imaging during extension work-up (e.g. several patients classified as cT3N+M1 were actually classified as pT3N0M1).

**Table 97** Correlation between cTNM, pTNM classifications.

| cTNM classification | Number | pTNM classification | Number |
|---|---|---|---|
| - | - | T0N0M1a | 01 (2,5 %) |
| - | - | T1N0M1a | 01 (2,5 %) |
| T2N0M1 | 02 (5%) | T2N0M1a | 01 (2,5 %) |
| T2N+M1 | 01 (2,5 %) | - | - |
| T3N0M1 | 03 (7,5 %) | T3N0M1a | 16 (40 %) |
| T3N+M1 | 34 (85 %) | $T3N_{1-2}M1a$ | 20 (50 %) |
| - | - | $T4N_{1-2}M1a$ | 01 (2,5 %) |
| Total | 40 (100 %) | Total | 40 (100 %) |

Starting in 2019, a new WHO classification of tumors (181) The histological types described are as follows:

| | |
|---|---|
| **Malignant epithelial tumours** | |
| 8140/3 | Adenocarcinoma NOS |
| 8213/3 | Serrated adenocarcinoma |
| 8262/3* | Adenoma-like adenocarcinoma |
| 8265/3 | Micropapillary adenocarcinoma |
| 8480/3 | Mucinous adenocarcinoma |
| 8490/3 | Poorly cohesive carcinoma |
| 8490/3 | Signet-ring cell carcinoma |
| 8510/3 | Medullary adenocarcinoma |
| 8560/3 | Adenosquamous carcinoma |
| 8020/3 | Carcinoma, undifferentiated, NOS |
| 8033/3* | Carcinoma with sarcomatoid component |

**Figure 64** Histological types in colorectal cancer according to the 2019 WHO tumor classification 5ème edition. (181).

## N. Recidivism:

Patient follow-up averaged 15 months, with a median of 12.5 months and extremes ranging from 2 months to 41 months.

During this period, 9 patients had a recurrence (22.5%), with a mean time to recurrence of 13.55 months . Seven times out of 9, the disease recurred in the liver. This recurrence was resectable in two patients. In the remaining 7 patients, drug therapy was initiated.

In a patient operated on for a left colonic tumour with a single liver metastasis, the recurrence was revealed by a single epiploic nodule that appeared at 13 months, confirmed on PET scan. This nodule was resected laparoscopically, and the anatomopathological study confirmed its carcinomatous nature. The patient was alive at 37 months without recurrence.

In our statistical analysis, only one variable was associated with recurrence: N+ cTNM classification ($p = 0.032$).

The hazard ratio was also high for the N+ of the pTNM classification, without the p being significant. (HR= 4.250) ($p = 0.088$).

This analysis could not be highly conclusive, given the lack of hindsight.

In the literature Takasu (162) over a follow-up period of 31.5 ± 33.5 months (0.6-95.2 months) reported a recurrence rate of 42.8% (liver or lung).

Ratti (146) in his comparative study, over a mean follow-up period of 37 months (15-75 months) reported a recurrence rate of 36% in the laparoscopic arm and 54% in the laparotomy arm, with a significant difference ($p = 0.04$).

In the laparoscopic arm, recurrence was hepatic in 44.4% of cases, extra-hepatic in 22.2% and mixed in 33.3%.

Recurrence was treated with re-resection in 22.2% of cases, radiofrequency in 11.1% and medication in 77.8%.

This recurrence and management profile is similar to that of our series, and the possibility of curative treatment of recurrence exists, but remains a minority.

In Xu's study (166)after 36 months' follow-up, the recurrence rate in the laparoscopy arm was 75%, compared with 70% in the laparotomy group.
Recurrence is therefore frequent in this situation of synchronous liver metastases, despite initial curative treatment.

## O. Survival:

As previously mentioned, the average follow-up period was 15 months, with a median of 12.5 months and extremes ranging from 2 months to 41 months.
Half of our workforce had been included in the study by 2019.
All patients in our study were alive at the cut-off date, but the follow-up was insufficient to comment on overall survival.
In contrast, mean recurrence-free survival was 28.91 months, with a median of 27 months in our series.
There was no difference in the recurrence-free survival curves of the different subgroups tested (gender, age, primary tumor location, lymph node infiltration, R0/R1 nature of surgery and CEA level). Ratti (174) identified poor long-term prognostic factors in his study; in his multivariate analysis, tumor stage, lymph node infiltration, number of metastases and postoperative complications were independent prognostic factors.
Some authors report median overall survival and recurrence-free survival, while others report overall or recurrence-free survival rates at 1, 3 and 5 years.
The following table summarizes the remote results of the main comparative studies cited in Moris's systematic review (159).

**Table 98** Remote outcomes of laparoscopic vs. conventional surgery (159).

| Authors | Followup (months), (range) | Adjuvant Chemotherapy (%) | Recurrence, n (%) | Overall survival (months), median | Disease-free survival (months), median | OS 1st/3rd/5th | DFS 1st/ 3rd/5th |
|---|---|---|---|---|---|---|---|
| Comparative studies (OSR vs LSR patients) | | | | | | | |
| Chen et al[24] (2011) | 45.3 (36-72) | 100 vs 100 | N/a | N/a | N/a | 77.8/38.9/0 vs 82.6/43.5/ 8.6 $P > 0.05$ | N/a |
| Hu et al[25] (2012) | (16-81) | 100 vs 100 | 2 (15.38) vs 2 (15.38) | N/a | N/a | 92/54/31 vs 92/ 55/27 $P > 0.05$ | N/a |
| Takasu et al[26] (2013) | 41.2 vs 31.5 $P = 0.56$ | 100 vs 42.8 $P = 0.02$ | 6 (85.7) vs 3 (42.8) | N/a | N/a | 100/N/a/41.7 vs 100/N/a/ 50 $P = 0.67$ | N/a |
| Jung et al[27] (2014) | N/a | N/a | N/a | N/a | N/a | N/a | N/a |
| Ratti et al[28] (2016) | 37 vs 37 | N/a | 27 (54) vs 9 (36) | 57 vs 60 $P = 0.19$ | 38 vs 43 $P = 0.05$ | N/a | N/a |
| Ivanecz et al[29] (2017) | 78 vs 24 $P = 0.001$ | 50 vs 20 $P = 0.35$ | 4 (40) vs 2 (20) | N/a | N/a | 100/90/80 vs 100/75/N/a $P = 0.842$ | 90/60/60 vs 100/57/Na $P = 0.724$ |
| Gorgun et al[30] (2017) | 24.2 vs 20.3 $P = 0.34$ | 80 vs 84.6 | 12 (41.3) vs 2 (14.2) $P = 0.08$ | 19.1 vs 24.3 $P = 0.1$ | 8.4 vs 10 $P = 0.028$ | N/a | N/a |
| Xu et al[31] (2017) | 27.5 vs 27.5 | 100 vs 100 | 14 (70) vs 15 (75) | N/a | N/a | N/a/58.3%/N/a vs N/a/56.3%/N/a $P = 0.788$ | N/a/36.6%/N/a vs N/a/ 31.6%/N/a $P = 0.607$ |

Abbreviations: DFS, disease-free survival; LSR, laparoscopic synchronous resection; N/a, not available; OS, overall survival; OSR, open synchronous resection.

Interpretation of remote survival results in these comparative studies suggests that there is no difference between the two approaches, with median survival and survival at 1, 3 and 5 years being equivalent.
In 2018, Chen (182) had published the long-term results of his comparative study, there was no difference in overall survival and recurrence-free survival at 1 and 3 years between the two groups (laparoscopy vs laparotomy) (table 99).

**Table 99** Long-term results of Chen series (182).

| | Laparoscopic (n = 15) | Open (n = 15) | p - value |
|---|---|---|---|
| Median follow (months) | 19 | 13 | 0.91 |
| Disease free | | | 0.99 |
| Mean (month) | 13 | 10 | |
| 1 year | 0.56 | 0.70 | |
| 3 year | 0.35 | 0.15 | |
| Overall survival | | | 0.14 |
| Mean (month) | 26 | 22 | |
| 1 year | 1.00 | 0.84 | |
| 3 year | 0.73 | 0.48 | |
| Adjuvant chemotherapy | 12 | 13 | |
| Recurrence | 8 | 8 | 1.00 |
| Death | 2 | 5 | 0.09 |
| Site of initial recurrence | | | 0.85 |
| Liver | 6 | 6 | |
| Lung | 1 | 1 | |
| Peritonium | 0 | 1 | |
| Adrenal gland | 1 | 0 | |

Remote oncological results therefore appear equivalent between the two types of approach (laparoscopy/laparotomy) in the combined treatment of colorectal cancers with synchronous liver metastases.

# IX. Limitations of our work :

The aim of our study was to evaluate the feasibility and safety of the laparoscopic approach in combined surgery for colorectal cancer with synchronous liver metastases.
The results concerning the judgment criteria for the main objective (morbidity <30%, mortality <5%, no increase in morbidity-mortality compared with the control arm) were in favor of the feasibility of laparoscopy in this situation.
Results concerning secondary objectives were also in favor of the laparoscopic approach, since the conversion rate was 7.5% (TConv < 15%), postoperative rehabilitation was satisfactory, as was the quality of carcinological excision at both tumor sites (primary and metastatic).
On the other hand, the evaluation of recurrence and survival rates could not be optimally carried out given the insufficient follow-up.

On the other hand, this is a single-center study on a limited sample, whose results reflect the activity of a single team over a limited period.

This is a prospective, two-arm comparative study. A review of the literature on the laparoscopic approach to patients with synchronous liver metastases did not identify any randomized studies on the subject, for obvious ethical reasons. Nevertheless, to compensate for this, authors have often compared combined laparoscopic surgery with combined conventional surgery on contemporary groups or retrospectively against historical series. We did not carry out this type of study for the sake of accuracy, as retrospective data collection under our conditions was likely to be incomplete. We opted for a comparison of combined laparoscopic surgery vs. laparoscopic colorectal surgery alone, as was done by Van Der Poel (38) and Bretagnol (18) to answer this question: "in the context of combined surgery, would adding a ″minor″ liver time increase morbi-mortality compared with laparoscopic colorectal surgery alone?"
This comparison was all the more feasible at our level, as laparoscopic colorectal surgery for cancer was routinely performed. Data were collected prospectively for both arms of the study.

In terms of surgical results, simultaneous laparoscopic approach to both tumour sites was used in 25% of patients, but hybrid surgery was the predominant procedure in our series, possibly due to the more frequent posterior location of liver metastases in our patients, This may be explained by the more frequent posterior localization of hepatic metastases in our patients, but also by the surgical team's degree of learning in laparoscopic hepatic surgery. Our experience in this field is beginner's level, and has improved over time, thanks in part to the development of laparoscopic hepatic surgery for other pathologies within the department.

# X. Outlook :

We consider this work as the beginning of a solution to be proposed to patients with MHSCCR, the laparoscopic approach allows both tumor sites to be approached with the least parietal trauma possible, it is in this sense that the ″tout laparoscopic″ approach will have to be developed in the future and this requires greater expertise in laparoscopic liver surgery.

This approach must be reproducible, and therefore extended to the whole department team (and of course to other surgical teams).

With this in mind, we envisage two teams working together on the same operation, one for the colorectal phase and a second for the liver phase. This would improve both immediate and carcinological results, by providing expertise for each stage of the operation, with a better distribution of the workload for procedures that can last 6 to 7 hours, as previously reported.

Worldwide, other applications of laparoscopic surgery in combined situations have been reported, such as laparoscopic major liver resections associated with colorectal resection (16). The use of robotic surgery has also been reported (183). A new approach was described in 2019 by Karoui (184) for patients requiring a major hepatic resection, known as "The "Short-Cut" Laparoscopic Reverse Approach", consists in performing both resections laparoscopically a few days apart, starting with the major hepatic time. This approach enables the oncological result (R0 resection) to be achieved in a limited timeframe, while avoiding the risks of simultaneous resection in this context of major or complex surgery.

# XI. Recommendations:

Appropriate patient selection for the simultaneous laparoscopic approach is of paramount importance. When considering minimally invasive combined resection for Stage IV CRC, the limitations of both the simultaneous and laparoscopic approaches must be taken into account.

Patient characteristics and tumour stage must be considered. Table 100 summarizes the absolute and relative contraindications to the combined laparoscopic approach.

**Table 100** Contraindications of simultaneous laparoscopic approach (121).

| absolute contraindications | relative contraindications |
|---|---|
| PS > 2 | BMI > 30 (G°R : D) |
| Poor prognosis | More than 3 synchronous MH (G°R : C) |
| Occlusive or perforated colorectal tumor | Need for major liver resection (> 3 segments) (G°R : C) |
| Unresectable extrahepatic metastases | Lesions in segments I,VII,VIII (G°R: C) |
| R0 unlikely | Extraperitoneal rectal tumor (G°R: C/D) |
| | Primary colorectal tumor > 5cm; (G°R: C/D) |

## XII. Conclusion:

The results of our study support the feasibility of laparoscopy in the management of colorectal cancer with synchronous liver metastases in selected patients.

In addition to its diagnostic value, laparoscopy can be used exclusively or in association with laparotomy for curative purposes in combined surgery, and can also constitute the first stage of ″down staging″ preparing for a major hepatectomy.

Minor liver surgery can be combined with laparoscopic colorectal surgery without increasing morbidity.

The quality of exeresis in the combined laparoscopic approach is good, but distant oncological results remain to be assessed.

# XIII. Bibliography :


1. Bray F, Ferlay J, Soerjomataram I, Siegel RL, Torre LA, Jemal A. Global cancer statistics 2018: GLOBOCAN estimates of incidence and mortality worldwide for 36 cancers in 185 countries. CA: A Cancer Journal for Clinicians. nov 2018;68(6):394-424.

2. Ferlay J, Colombet M, Soerjomataram I, Mathers C, Parkin DM, Piñeros M, et al. Estimating the global cancer incidence and mortality in 2018: GLOBOCAN sources and methods. Int J Cancer. 15 Apr 2019;144(8):1941-53.

3. Ferlay J, Ervik M, Lam F, Colombet M, Mery L, Piñeros M, Znaor A, Soerjomataram I, Bray F. Cancer today [Internet]. [cited 13 Feb 2020]. Available from: http://gco.iarc.fr/today/home

4. Zitouni M et al. 2015-2019 national cancer plan. ANDS October 2014;

5. Hammouda PD, N AHN, Boutekdjiret L, Lalaoui R, Kadri C. Registre des Tumeurs de la wilaya d'Alger. 2017;33.

6. Siegel R, DeSantis C, Jemal A. Colorectal cancer statistics, 2014: Colorectal Cancer Statistics, 2014. CA A Cancer Journal for Clinicians. march 2014;64(2):104-17.

7. Clark ME, Smith RR. Liver-directed therapies in metastatic colorectal cancer. Journal of Gastrointestinal Oncology. 2014;5(5):14.

8. Martin RCG, Augenstein V, Reuter NP, Scoggins CR, McMasters KM. Simultaneous Versus Staged Resection for Synchronous Colorectal Cancer Liver Metastases. Journal of the American College of Surgeons. May 2009;208(5):842-50.

9. Schlag P, Hohenberger P, Herfarth C. Resection of liver metastases in colorectal cancer-competitive analysis of treatment results in synchronous versus metachronous metastases. Eur J Surg Oncol. August 1990;16(4):360-5.

10. Polignano FM, Quyn AJ, Sanjay P, Henderson NA, Tait IS. Totally laparoscopic strategies for the management of colorectal cancer with synchronous liver metastasis. Surg Endosc. Sept 2012;26(9):2571-8.

11. Mentha G, Majno PE, Andres A, Rubbia-Brandt L, Morel P, Roth AD. Neoadjuvant chemotherapy and resection of advanced synchronous liver metastases before treatment of the colorectal primary. Br J Surg. Jul 2006;93(7):872-8.

12. Demicheli R, Retsky MW, Hrushesky WJM, Baum M, Gukas ID. The effects of surgery on tumor growth: a century of investigations. Annals of Oncology. Nov 2008;19(11):1821-8.

13. Hillingsø JG, Wille-Jørgensen P. Staged or simultaneous resection of synchronous liver metastases from colorectal cancer - a systematic review. Colorectal Disease. Jan 2009;11(1):3-10.

14. Chen J, Li Q, Wang C, Zhu H, Shi Y, Zhao G. Simultaneous vs. staged resection for synchronous colorectal liver metastases: a metaanalysis. Int J Colorectal Dis. Feb 2011;26(2):191-9.

15. Nordlinger B, Guiguet M, Vaillant JC, Balladur P, Boudjema K, Bachellier P, et al. Surgical resection of colorectal carcinoma metastases to the liver. A prognostic scoring system to improve case selection, based on 1568 patients. Association Française de Chirurgie. Cancer. Apr 1, 1996;77(7):1254-62.

16. Tranchart H, Diop PS, Lainas P, Pourcher G, Catherine L, Franco D, et al. Laparoscopic major hepatectomy can be safely performed with colorectal surgery for synchronous colorectal liver metastasis. HPB. Jan 2011;13(1):46-50.

17. Brouquet A, Mortenson MM, Vauthey J-N, Rodriguez-Bigas MA, Overman MJ, Chang GJ, et al. Surgical Strategies for Synchronous Colorectal Liver Metastases in 156 Consecutive Patients: Classic, Combined or Reverse Strategy? Journal of the American College of Surgeons. June 2010;210(6):934-41.

18. Bretagnol F, Hatwell C, Farges O, Alves A, Belghiti J, Panis Y. Benefit of laparoscopy for rectal resection in patients operated simultaneously for synchronous liver metastases: Preliminary experience. Surgery. Sept 2008;144(3):436-41.

19. Martin R, Paty P, Fong Y, Grace A, Cohen A, DeMatteo R, et al. Simultaneous liver and colorectal resections are safe for synchronous colorectal liver metastasis. Journal of the American College of Surgeons. August 2003;197(2):233-41.

20. De Haas RJ, Adam R, Wicherts DA, Azoulay D, Bismuth H, Vibert E, et al. Comparison of simultaneous or delayed liver surgery for limited synchronous colorectal metastases. Br J Surg. August 2010;97(8):1279-89.

21. Reddy SK, Pawlik TM, Zorzi D, Gleisner AL, Ribero D, Assumpcao L, et al. Simultaneous Resections of Colorectal Cancer and Synchronous Liver Metastases: A Multi-institutional Analysis. Ann Surg Oncol. Nov 14, 2007;14(12):3481-91.

22. Guillou PJ, Quirke P, Thorpe H, Walker J, Jayne DG, Smith AM, et al. Short-term endpoints of conventional versus laparoscopic-assisted surgery in patients with colorectal cancer (MRC CLASICC trial): multicentre, randomised controlled trial. The Lancet. May 2005;365(9472):1718-26.

23. Lacy AM, García-Valdecasas JC, Delgado S, Castells A, Taurá P, Piqué JM, et al. Laparoscopy-assisted colectomy versus open colectomy for treatment of non-metastatic colon cancer: a randomised trial. The Lancet. June 2002;359(9325):2224-9.

24. Gagner M, Rheault M, Dubuc J. Laparoscopic partial hepatectomy for liver tumor. Surg Endosc 1992;6:99.

25. Topal B, Tiek J, Fieuws S, Aerts R, Van Cutsem E, Roskams T, et al. Minimally invasive liver surgery for metastases from colorectal cancer: oncologic outcome and prognostic factors. Surg Endosc. August 2012;26(8):2288-98.

26. Nguyen KT, Gamblin TC, Geller DA. World Review of Laparoscopic Liver Resection-2,804 Patients: Annals of Surgery. nov 2009;250(5):831-41.

27. Kim Y, Kim BR, Kim IY, Kim HS. Differences in clinical features between laparoscopy and open resection for primary tumor in patients with stage IV colorectal cancer. OTT. nov 2015;3441.

28. Geiger TM, Tebb ZD, Sato E, Miedema BW, Awad ZT. Laparoscopic Resection of Colon Cancer and Synchronous Liver Metastasis. Journal of Laparoendoscopic & Advanced Surgical Techniques. Feb 2006;16(1):51-3.

29. Leung KL, Lee JFY, Yiu RYC, Ng SSM, Li JCM. Simultaneous Laparoscopic Resection of Rectal Cancer and Liver Metastasis. Journal of Laparoendoscopic & Advanced Surgical Techniques. oct 2006;16(5):486-8.

30. Hatwell C, Bretagnol F, Farges O, Belghiti J, Panis Y. Laparoscopic resection of colorectal cancer facilitates simultaneous surgery of synchronous liver metastases. Colorectal Disease. Jan 2013;15(1):e21-8.

31. Huh JW, Koh YS, Kim HR, Cho CK, Kim YJ. Comparison of laparoscopic and open colorectal resections for patients undergoing simultaneous R0 resection for liver metastases. Surg Endosc. Jan 2011;25(1):193-8.

32. Ratti F, Catena M, Di Palo S, Staudacher C, Aldrighetti L. Laparoscopic Approach for Primary Colorectal Cancer Improves Outcome of Patients Undergoing Combined Open Hepatic Resection for Liver Metastases. World J Surg. oct 2015;39(10):2573-82.

33. Jung KU, Kim HC, Cho YB, Kwon CHD, Yun SH, Heo JS, et al. Outcomes of Simultaneous Laparoscopic Colorectal and Hepatic Resection for Patients with Colorectal Cancers: A Comparative Study. Journal of Laparoendoscopic & Advanced Surgical Techniques. apr 2014;24(4):229-35.

34. Lupinacci RM, Andraus W, De Paiva Haddad LB, Carneiro D'Albuquerque LA, Herman P. Simultaneous laparoscopic resection of primary colorectal cancer and associated liver metastases: a systematic review. Tech Coloproctol. Feb 2014;18(2):129-35.

35. Ferretti S, Tranchart H, Buell JF, Eretta C, Patriti A, Spampinato MG, et al. Laparoscopic Simultaneous Resection of Colorectal Primary Tumor and Liver Metastases: Results of a Multicenter International Study. World J Surg. August 2015;39(8):2052-60.

36. Tranchart H, Fuks D, Vigano L, Ferretti S, Paye F, Wakabayashi G, et al. Laparoscopic simultaneous resection of colorectal primary tumor and liver metastases: a propensity score matching analysis. Surg Endosc. May 2016;30(5):1853-62.

37. Garritano S, Selvaggi F, Spampinato MG. Simultaneous Minimally Invasive Treatment of Colorectal Neoplasm with Synchronous Liver Metastasis. BioMed Research International. 2016;2016:1-7.

38. Van der Poel MJ, Tanis PJ, Marsman HA, Rijken AM, Gertsen EC, Ovaere S, et al. Laparoscopic combined resection of liver metastases and colorectal cancer: a multicenter, case-matched study using propensity scores. Surg Endosc. Apr 2019;33(4):1124-30.

39. Pessaux P, Panaro F. Advantages of the first-step totally laparoscopic approach in 2-staged hepatectomy for colorectal synchronous liver metastasis. Surgery. Apr 2009;145(4):453.

40. Emile J-F, Leteurtre E, Guyétant S. Natural history of cancer. Collège Français des Pathologistes (CoPath); 2011.

41. Paschos KA. Natural history of hepatic metastases from colorectal cancer - pathobiological pathways with clinical significance. WJG. 2014;20(14):3719.

42. Tougeron D. Colorectal carcinogenesis, fundamental data. In: EM-Consulte [Internet]. Elsevier Masson; [cited 2020 Feb 21]. Available from: https://www.em-consulte.com/article/905231/carcinogenese-colorectale-donnees-fondamentales

43. Karoui M, Tresallet C, Brouquet A, Radvanyi H, Penna C. Colorectal carcinogenesis. Mise au point. 2007;6.

44. Worthley DL, Leggett BA. Colorectal Cancer: Molecular Features and Clinical Opportunities. Colorectal Cancer. :8.

45. McDonald SA, Preston SL, Lovell MJ, Wright NA, Jankowski JA. Mechanisms of Disease: from stem cells to colorectal cancer. Nat Rev Gastroenterol Hepatol. May 2006;3(5):267-74.

46. Hisabe T, Hirai F, Matsui T. Development and progression of colorectal cancer based on follow-up analysis: Natural history of colorectal cancer. Digestive Endoscopy. Apr 2014;26:73-7.

47. Jones S, Chen W -d., Parmigiani G, Diehl F, Beerenwinkel N, Antal T, et al. Comparative lesion sequencing provides insights into tumor evolution. Proceedings of the National Academy of Sciences. March 18, 2008;105(11):4283-8.

48. Bouvier A-M, Manfredi S, Lejeune C. The natural history of colorectal cancer revisited. 2019;6.

49. Agnes N. Colonic carcinogenesis: molecular subtyping of the early stages of non-MIN phenotype colon cancer. :137.

50. Fearon ER, Vogelstein B. A genetic model for colorectal tumorigenesis. Cell. June 1990;61(5):759-67.

51. Olschwang S, Paraf F, Laurent-Puig P, Wang Q, Lecuru F, Hamelin R, et al. Recent contributions to the identification and screening of Lynch syndrome. Gastroentérologie Clinique et Biologique. Feb 2007;31(2):136-40.

52. Phelip JM, Tougeron D, Léonard D, Benhaim L, Desolneux G, Dupré A, et al. Metastatic colorectal cancer (mCRC): French intergroup clinical practice guidelines for diagnosis, treatments and follow-up (SNFGE, FFCD, GERCOR, UNICANCER, SFCD, SFED, SFRO, SFR). Digestive and Liver Disease. oct 2019;51(10):1357-63.

53. Guinney J, Dienstmann R, Wang X, de Reyniès A, Schlicker A, Soneson C, et al. The consensus molecular subtypes of colorectal cancer. Nat Med. nov 2015;21(11):1350-6.

54. Gallot D. Surgical anatomy of the colon. EMC - Techniques chirurgicales - Appareil digestif. Jan 2006;1(2):1-8.

55. Beaugerie L, Sokol H. Les fondamentaux-pathologie-digestive_octobre-2014. Elsevier-Masson; 2014.

56. Heald RJ, Husband EM, Ryall RDH. The mesorectum in rectal cancer surgery-the clue to pelvic recurrence? Br J Surg. Oct 1982;69(10):613-6.

57. Fléjou J-F, Cervera P. Anatomie pathologique : en marche vers l'analyse moléculaire. Gastroentérologie Clinique et Biologique. August 2009;33(8-9):767-74.

58. Pickhardt PJ, Pooler BD, Kim DH, Hassan C, Matkowskyj KA, Halberg RB. The natural history of colorectal polyps. Gastroenterology Clinics of North America. sept 2018;47(3):515-36.

59. Bosman FT, World Health Organization, International Agency for Research on Cancer, editors. WHO classification of tumours of the digestive system. 4th ed. Lyon: International Agency for Research on Cancer; 2010. 417 p. (World Health Organization classification of tumours).

60. Mäkinen MJ. Colorectal serrated adenocarcinoma. Histopathology. Jan 2007;50(1):131-50.

61. Sedkaoui C. DESM thesis chemotherapy and targeted therapy in metastatic colorectal cancer. 2015.

62. Brierley J, Gospodarowicz MK, Wittekind C, editors. TNM classification of malignant tumours. Eighth edition. Chichester, West Sussex, UK; Hoboken, NJ: John Wiley & Sons, Inc; 2017.

63. Bibeau F, Goldman-Levy G. Colorectal cancer: typical pathology report in 2014. Oncology. dec 2014;16(11-12):525-36.

64. Quirke P, Morris E. Reporting colorectal cancer. Histopathology. Jan 2007;50(1):103-12.

65. Dworak O, Keilholz L, Hoffmann A. Pathological features of rectal cancer after preoperative radiochemotherapy. :5.

66. Rubbia-Brandt L, Giostra E, Brezault C, Roth AD, Andres A, Audard V, et al. Importance of histological tumor response assessment in predicting the outcome in patients with colorectal liver metastases treated with neo-adjuvant chemotherapy followed by liver surgery. Annals of Oncology. Feb 2007;18(2):299-304.

67. Lugli A, Karamitopoulou E, Zlobec I. Tumour budding: a promising parameter in colorectal cancer. Br J Cancer. May 2012;106(11):1713-7.

68. Bibeau F, Rivière B, Boissière F, Jourdan M-F, Bodin X, Perrault V, et al. Management of liver metastases of colorectal origin after induction therapy. Place du pathologiste en 2011. Annales de Pathologie. Dec 2011;31(6):427-32.

69. Mandard AM, Dalibard F, Mandard JC, Marnay J, Henry-Amar M, Petiot JF, et al. Pathologic assessment of tumor regression after preoperative chemoradiotherapy of esophageal carcinoma. Clinicopathologic correlations. Cancer. June 1, 1994;73(11):2680-6.

70. Maru DM, Kopetz S, Boonsirikamchai P, Agarwal A, Chun YS, Wang H, et al. Tumor Thickness at the Tumor-normal Interface: A Novel Pathologic Indicator of Chemotherapy Response in Hepatic Colorectal Metastases: The American Journal of Surgical Pathology. sept 2010;34(9):1287-94.

71. Mentha G, Terraz S, Morel P, Andres A, Giostra E, Roth A, et al. Dangerous halo after neoadjuvant chemotherapy and two-step hepatectomy for colorectal liver metastases. Br J Surg. Jan 2009;96(1):95-103.

72. Vauthey J-N, Pawlik TM, Ribero D, Wu T-T, Zorzi D, Hoff PM, et al. Chemotherapy Regimen Predicts Steatohepatitis and an Increase in 90-Day Mortality After Surgery for Hepatic Colorectal Metastases. JCO. May 1, 2006;24(13):2065-72.

73. Rubbia-Brandt L, Lauwers GY, Wang H, Majno PE, Tanabe K, X Zhu A, et al. Sinusoidal obstruction syndrome and nodular regenerative hyperplasia are frequent oxaliplatin-associated liver lesions and partially prevented by bevacizumab in patients with hepatic colorectal metastasis. Histopathology. March 2010;56(4):430-9.

74. Hermanek P, Wittekind C. Residual tumor (R) classification and prognosis. Semin Surg Oncol. Jan 1994;10(1):12-20.

75. Sternberg A, Amar M, Alfici R, Groisman G. Conclusions from a study of venous invasion in stage IV colorectal adenocarcinoma. Journal of Clinical Pathology. 1 Jan 2002;55(1):17-21.

76. Liebig C, Ayala G, Wilks J, Verstovsek G, Liu H, Agarwal N, et al. Perineural Invasion Is an Independent Predictor of Outcome in Colorectal Cancer. JCO. Nov 1, 2009;27(31):5131-7.

77. Fujita S, Shimoda T, Yoshimura K, Yamamoto S, Akasu T, Moriya Y. Prospective evaluation of prognostic factors in patients with colorectal cancer undergoing curative resection. J Surg Oncol. Nov 2003;84(3):127-31.

78. French AJ, Sargent DJ, Burgart LJ, Foster NR, Kabat BF, Goldberg R, et al. Prognostic Significance of Defective Mismatch Repair and BRAF V600E in Patients with Colon Cancer. Clinical Cancer Research. June 1, 2008;14(11):3408-15.

79. Bibeau F, Frugier H, Pedot M, Boissière-Michot F. Microsatellite instability in colorectal cancer. Oncology. sept 2012;14(9):525-9.

80. Samowitz WS, Sweeney C, Herrick J, Albertsen H, Levin TR, Murtaugh MA, et al. Poor Survival Associated with the *BRAF* V600E Mutation in Microsatellite-Stable Colon Cancers. Cancer Res. 15 Jul 2005;65(14):6063-9.

81. Douillard J-Y, Oliner KS, Siena S, Tabernero J, Burkes R, Barugel M, et al. Panitumumab-FOLFOX4 Treatment and *RAS* Mutations in Colorectal Cancer. N Engl J Med. Sep 12, 2013;369(11):1023-34.

82. Lecomte T, André T, Bibeau F, Blanc B, Cohen R, Lagasse JP,, Laurent-Puig P, Martin-Babau J, Panis Y, Portales F, Taïeb J, Vaillant E. Non-metastatic colon cancer. Thésaurus National de Cancérologie Digestive. [Internet]. 2019. Available at: https://www.snfge.org/tncd and http://www.tncd.org

83. Gönen M, Schrag D, Weiser MR. Nodal Staging Score: A Tool to Assess Adequate Staging of Node-Negative Colon Cancer. JCO. 2009 Dec 20;27(36):6166-71.

84. Wu Z, Qin G, Zhao N, Jia H, Zheng X. Assessing the adequacy of lymph node yield for different tumor stages of colon cancer by nodal staging scores. BMC Cancer. dec 2017;17(1):498.

85. Nagtegaal ID, Knijn N, Hugen N, Marshall HC, Sugihara K, Tot T, et al. Tumor Deposits in Colorectal Cancer: Improving the Value of Modern Staging-A Systematic Review and Meta-Analysis. JCO. Apr 1, 2017;35(10):1119-27.

86. Cotte E, Artru P, Christou N, Conroy T, Doyen J, Fabre J, Legoux JL, Hoeffel C, Léonard D,, Meillan N, Paix A, Pioche M, Rivin Del Campo E, Vendrely V. "Cancer du rectum". Thésaurus National de Cancérologie Digestive, March 2019 [Internet]. 2019. Available from: http://www.tncd.org

87. Gallix B. What examinations should be performed in the pretherapeutic extension workup? Critères de qualité et résultats attendus. /data/revues/03998320/00270HS2/25/ [Internet]. 2008 Feb 29 [cited 2020 Feb 22]; Available from: https://www.em-consulte.com/en/article/99681

88. Ong KO, Leen E. Radiological staging of colorectal liver metastases. Surgical Oncology. Jul 2007;16(1):7-14.

89. Albrecht T, Blomley MJK, Burns PN, Wilson S, Harvey CJ, Leen E, et al. Improved Detection of Hepatic Metastases with Pulse-Inversion US during the Liver-specific Phase of SHU 508A: Multicenter Study. Radiology. May 2003;227(2):361-70.

90. Nordlinger B, Jaeck D. Multidisciplinary treatment. Bulletin de l'Académie Nationale de Médecine. feb 2015;199(2-3):213-22.

91. Zalinski S, Mariette C, Farges O. Prise en charge des patients atteints de métastases hépatiques synchrones du cancer colorectal. Recommandations pour la Pratique Clinique. Recommendations of the French Society of Digestive Surgery (SFCD) and the Association of Hepatobiliary Surgery and Liver Transplantation (ACHBT). Short text. Journal de Chirurgie Viscérale. June 2011;148(3):196-208.

92. Nordlinger B, Sorbye H, Glimelius B, Poston GJ, Schlag PM, Rougier P, et al. Perioperative chemotherapy with FOLFOX4 and surgery versus surgery alone for resectable liver metastases from colorectal cancer (EORTC Intergroup trial 40983): a randomised controlled trial. The Lancet. March 2008;371(9617):1007-16.

93. Nordlinger B, Sorbye H, Glimelius B, Poston GJ, Schlag PM, Rougier P, et al. Perioperative FOLFOX4 chemotherapy and surgery versus surgery alone for resectable liver metastases from colorectal cancer (EORTC 40983): long-term results of a randomised, controlled, phase 3 trial. The Lancet Oncology. nov 2013;14(12):1208-15.

94. Nordlinger B, Van Cutsem E, Gruenberger T, Glimelius B, Poston G, Rougier P, et al. Combination of surgery and chemotherapy and the role of targeted agents in the treatment of patients with colorectal liver metastases: recommendations from an expert panel. Annals of Oncology. June 2009;20(6):985-92.

95. Schwartzberg LS, Rivera F, Karthaus M, Fasola G, Canon J-L, Hecht JR, et al. PEAK: A Randomized, Multicenter Phase II Study of Panitumumab Plus Modified Fluorouracil, Leucovorin, and Oxaliplatin (mFOLFOX6) or Bevacizumab Plus mFOLFOX6 in Patients With Previously Untreated, Unresectable, Wild-Type *KRAS* Exon 2 Metastatic Colorectal Cancer. JCO. 20 Jul 2014;32(21):2240-7.

96. Hubert C, Gigot J-F. Surgical treatment of colorectal liver metastases. Bulletin du Cancer. March 1, 2008;95(3):365-8.

97. Cunningham D, Lang I, Marcuello E, Lorusso V, Ocvirk J, Shin DB, et al. Bevacizumab plus capecitabine versus capecitabine alone in elderly patients with previously untreated metastatic colorectal cancer (AVEX): an open-label, randomised phase 3 trial. The Lancet Oncology. oct 2013;14(11):1077-85.

98. Adam R, de Gramont A, Figueras J, Kokudo N, Kunstlinger F, Loyer E, et al. Managing synchronous liver metastases from colorectal cancer: A multidisciplinary international consensus. Cancer Treatment Reviews. nov 2015;41(9):729-41.

99. Brouquet A, Benoist S. Which therapeutic strategy in rectal cancer with synchronous liver metastases: Question 8. Colon Rectum. may 2012;6(2):105-13.

100. Bosset J-F, Collette L, Calais G, Mineur L, Maingon P, Radosevic-Jelic L, et al. Chemotherapy with Preoperative Radiotherapy in Rectal Cancer. N Engl J Med. Sep 14, 2006;355(11):1114-23.

101. G Manceau, Benoist G, Bachet JB. What is the evolution of synchronous liver metastases during radiochemotherapy for locally advanced rectal cancer? 2009;15.

102. Karoui M, Vigano L, Goyer P, Ferrero A, Luciani A, Aglietta M, et al. Combined first-stage hepatectomy and colorectal resection in a two-stage hepatectomy strategy for bilobar synchronous liver metastases. Br J Surg. 5 Jul 2010;97(9):1354-62.

103. Brouquet A, Abdalla EK, Kopetz S, Garrett CR, Overman MJ, Eng C, et al. High Survival Rate After Two-Stage Resection of Advanced Colorectal Liver Metastases: Response-Based Selection and Complete Resection Define Outcome. JCO. March 10, 2011;29(8):1083-90.

104. Van der Pool AE, de Wilt JH, Lalmahomed ZS, Eggermont AM, IJzermans JN, Verhoef C. Optimizing the outcome of surgery in patients with rectal cancer and synchronous liver metastases. Br J Surg. March 2010;97(3):383-90.

105. Strasberg SM, Belghiti J, Clavien P-A, Gadzijev E, Garden JO, Lau W-Y, et al. The Brisbane 2000 Terminology of Liver Anatomy and Resections. HPB. 2000;2(3):333-9.

106. Kooby DA, Stockman J, Ben-Porat L, Gonen M, Jarnagin WR, Dematteo RP, et al. Influence of Transfusions on Perioperative and Long-Term Outcome in Patients Following Hepatic Resection for Colorectal Metastases: Annals of Surgery. June 2003;237(6):860-70.

107. Squires MH, Kooby DA, Poultsides GA, Weber SM, Bloomston M, Fields RC, et al. Effect of Perioperative Transfusion on Recurrence and Survival after Gastric Cancer Resection: A 7-Institution Analysis of 765 Patients from the US Gastric Cancer Collaborative. Journal of the American College of Surgeons. sept 2015;221(3):767-77.

108. Ambiru S, Miyazaki M, Isono T, Ito H, Nakagawa K, Shimizu H, et al. Hepatic resection for colorectal metastases: Analysis of prognostic factors. Diseases of the Colon & Rectum. May 1999;42(5):632-9.

109. Kokudo N, Miki Y, Sugai S, Yanagisawa A, Kato Y, Sakamoto Y, et al. Genetic and Histological Assessment of Surgical Margins in Resected Liver Metastases From Colorectal Carcinoma: Minimum Surgical Margins for Successful Resection. Arch Surg [Internet]. 1 Jul 2002 [cited 28 Feb 2020];137(7). Available from: http://archsurg.jamanetwork.com/article.aspx?doi=10.1001/archsurg.137.7.833

110. Chiche L. Which liver metastases are resectable from the start /data/revues/03998320/00270HS2/41/ [Internet]. 29 Feb 2008 [cited 25 March 2020]; Available from: https://www.em-consulte.com/en/article/99682

111. Chang SB. Modified Makuuchi Incision for Foregut Procedures. Arch Surg. March 1, 2010;145(3):281.

112. Grant A, Neuberger J. Guidelines on the use of liver biopsy in clinical practice. British Society of Gastroenterology. Gut. Oct 1999;45 Suppl 4:IV1-11.

113. Federation of Visceral and Digestive Surgery. Risks associated with the creation of pneumoperitoneum. Solutions for patient safety. Journal of Visceral Surgery. march 2012;149(2):1-9.

114. Wakabayashi G. What has changed after the Morioka consensus conference 2014 on laparoscopic liver resection? Hepatobiliary Surg Nutr. August 2016;5(4):281-9.

115. Abu Hilal M, Aldrighetti L, Dagher I, Edwin B, Troisi RI, Alikhanov R, et al. The Southampton Consensus Guidelines for Laparoscopic Liver Surgery: From Indication to Implementation. Annals of Surgery. july 2018;268(1):11-8.

116. Fretland ÅA, Dagenborg VJ, Bjørnelv GMW, Kazaryan AM, Kristiansen R, Fagerland MW, et al. Laparoscopic Versus Open Resection for Colorectal Liver Metastases: The OSLO-COMET Randomized Controlled Trial. Annals of Surgery. feb 2018;267(2):199-207.

117. Halls MC, Berardi G, Cipriani F, Barkhatov L, Lainas P, Harris S, et al. Development and validation of a difficulty score to predict intraoperative complications during laparoscopic liver resection: Difficulty score to predict complications during laparoscopic liver resection. Br J Surg. August 2018;105(9):1182-91.

118. Ciria R, Ayllon MD, Briceño J. Difficulty scores in laparoscopic liver surgery-getting closer to a powerful and necessary tool. Hepatobiliary Surg Nutr. August 2019;8(4):428-30.

119. Samama C-M, Gafsou B, Jeandel T, Laporte S, Steib A, Marret E, et al. Prevention of postoperative venous thromboembolic disease. Updated 2011. Short text. Annales Françaises d'Anesthésie et de Réanimation. Dec 2011;30(12):947-51.

120. Martin C, Auboyer C, Boisson M, Dupont H, Gauzit R, Kitzis M, et al. Antibioprophylaxis in surgery and interventional medicine (adult patients). Update 2017. Anaesthesia Critical Care & Pain Medicine. oct 2019;38(5):549-62.

121. Calise F, Casciola L. Minimally invasive surgery of the liver. New York: Springer; 2012.

122. Bateman AC, Jaynes E, Bateman AR. Rectal cancer staging post neoadjuvant therapy - how should the changes be assessed? Histopathology. May 2009;54(6):713-21.

123 Kazaryan AM, Røsok BI, Edwin B. Morbidity Assessment in Surgery: Refinement Proposal Based on a Concept of Perioperative Adverse Events. ISRN Surgery. 2013;2013:1-7.

124. Satava RM. Identification and reduction of surgical error using simulation. Minimally Invasive Therapy & Allied Technologies. Jan 2005;14(4-5):257-61.

125. Dindo D, Demartines N, Clavien P-A. Classification of Surgical Complications: A New Proposal With Evaluation in a Cohort of 6336 Patients and Results of a Survey. Annals of Surgery. August 2004;240(2):205-13.

126. Clavien PA, Barkun J, de Oliveira ML, Vauthey JN, Dindo D, Schulick RD, et al. The Clavien-Dindo Classification of Surgical Complications: Five-Year Experience. Annals of Surgery. August 2009;250(2):187-96.

127. Slankamenac K, Graf R, Barkun J, Puhan MA, Clavien P-A. The Comprehensive Complication Index: A Novel Continuous Scale to Measure Surgical Morbidity. Annals of Surgery. july 2013;258(1):1-7.

128. Katayama H, Kurokawa Y, Nakamura K, Ito H, Kanemitsu Y, Masuda N, et al. Extended Clavien-Dindo classification of surgical complications: Japan Clinical Oncology Group postoperative complications criteria. Surg Today. June 2016;46(6):668-85.

129. Bentabak K, Boubnider M, Feraoun S, Oukkal M, Oukrif S, Terki N. Manuel de Prise en Charge Du Cancer du Rectum. 2016.

130. Floriani I, Torri V, Rulli E, Garavaglia D, Compagnoni A, Salvolini L, et al. Performance of imaging modalities in diagnosis of liver metastases from colorectal cancer: A systematic review and meta-analysis: Radiological Evaluation of Liver Metastases. J Magn Reson Imaging. Jan 2010;31(1):19-31.

131. Andres A, Toso C, Adam R, Barroso E, Hubert C, Capussotti L, et al. A Survival Analysis of the Liver-First Reversed Management of Advanced Simultaneous Colorectal Liver Metastases: A LiverMetSurvey-Based Study. Annals of Surgery. nov 2012;256(5):772-9.

132. Mentha G, Roth AD, Terraz S, Giostra E, Gervaz P, Andres A, et al. 'Liver First' Approach in the Treatment of Colorectal Cancer with Synchronous Liver Metastases. Dig Surg. 2008;25(6):430-5.

133. Fahy BN, Fischer CP. Synchronous resection of colorectal primary and hepatic metastasis. Journal of Gastrointestinal Oncology. 2012;3(1):11.

134. Ihnát P, Vávra P, Zonča P. Treatment strategies for colorectal carcinoma with synchronous liver metastases: Which way to go? WJG. June 14, 2015;21(22):7014-21.

135. Lykoudis PM, O'Reilly D, Nastos K, Fusai G. Systematic review of surgical management of synchronous colorectal liver metastases. Br J Surg. May 2014;101(6):605-12.

136. Lyass S, Zamir G, Matot I, Goitein D, Eid A, Jurim O. Combined colon and hepatic resection for synchronous colorectal liver metastases. J Surg Oncol. Sept 2001;78(1):17-21.

137. Weber JC, Bachellier P, Oussoultzoglou E, Jaeck D. Simultaneous resection of colorectal primary tumour and synchronous liver metastases. Br J Surg. August 2003;90(8):956-62.

138. Li Z, Liu K, Duan J, Li Z, Su C, Yang J. Meta-analysis of simultaneous versus staged resection for synchronous colorectal liver metastases: Synchronous colorectal liver metastases. Hepatology Research. Jan 2013;43(1):72-83.

139. Jacobs M, Verdeja JC, Goldstein HS. Minimally invasive colon resection (laparoscopic colectomy). Surg Laparosc Endosc. Sept 1991;1(3):144-50.

140. Alexander RJT, Jaques BC, Mitchell KG. Laparoscopically assisted colectomy and wound recurrence. The Lancet. Jan 1993;341(8839):249-50.

141. Hughes ES, McDermott FT, Polglase AL, Johnson WR. Tumor recurrence in the abdominal wall scar tissue after large-bowel cancer surgery. Dis Colon Rectum. Sept 1983;26(9):571-2.

142. Reilly WT, Nelson H, Schroeder G, Wieand HS, Bolton J, O'Connell MJ. Wound recurrence following conventional treatment of colorectal cancer. A rare but perhaps underestimated problem. Dis Colon Rectum. Feb 1996;39(2):200-7.

143. Hahnloser D, Hetzer F, Lesurtel M, Demartines N, Clavien P-A. Laparoscopic resection for all colon cancers? Swiss Medical Journal. 2004;

144. Morneau M, Boulanger J, Charlebois P, Latulippe J-F, Lougnarath R, Thibault C, et al. Laparoscopic versus open surgery for the treatment of colorectal cancer: a literature review and recommendations from the Comité de l'évolution des pratiques en oncologie. Can J Surg. Oct 1, 2013;56(5):297-310.

145. Lin C, Lu S, Tang C, Sheng Q, Pan Z, Chen W, et al. Simultaneous Resection of Colorectal Cancer and Liver Metastases through Hand-assisted Laparoscopic Surgery: Preliminary Exploration. Hepatogastroenterology. june 2014;61(132):1014-7.

146. Ratti F, Catena M, Di Palo S, Staudacher C, Aldrighetti L. Impact of totally laparoscopic combined management of colorectal cancer with synchronous hepatic metastases on severity of complications: a propensity-score-based analysis. Surg Endosc. nov 2016;30(11):4934-45.

147. Patriti A, Ceccarelli G, Bartoli A, Spaziani A, Lapalorcia LM, Casciola L. Laparoscopic and robot-assisted one-stage resection of colorectal cancer with synchronous liver metastases: a pilot study. J Hepatobiliary Pancreat Surg. Jul 2009;16(4):450-7.

148. Kim Y, Kim BR, Kim IY, Kim HS. Differences in clinical features between laparoscopy and open resection for primary tumor in patients with stage IV colorectal cancer. OTT. nov 2015;3441.

149. Yamashita S, Sakamoto Y, Yamamoto S, Takemura N, Omichi K, Shinkawa H, et al. Efficacy of Preoperative Portal Vein Embolization Among Patients with Hepatocellular Carcinoma, Biliary Tract Cancer, and Colorectal Liver Metastases: A Comparative Study Based on Single-Center Experience of 319 Cases. Ann Surg Oncol. June 2017;24(6):1557-68.

150. Robles R, Marín C, Lopez-Conesa A, Capel A, Perez-Flores D, Parrilla P. Comparative study of right portal vein ligation versus embolisation for induction of hypertrophy in two-stage hepatectomy for multiple bilateral colorectal liver metastases. European Journal of Surgical Oncology (EJSO). july 2012;38(7):586-93.

151. Biggemann L, Uhlig J, Streit U, Sack H, Guo XC, Jung C, et al. Future liver remnant growth after various portal vein embolization regimens: a quantitative comparison. Minimally Invasive Therapy & Allied Technologies. march 2019;1-9.

152. Van den Esschert JW, van Lienden KP, de Graaf W, Maas MAW, Roelofs JJTH, Heger M, et al. Portal vein embolization induces more liver regeneration than portal vein ligation in a standardized rabbit model. Surgery. March 2011;149(3):378-85.

153. Capussotti L. Portal Vein Ligation as an Efficient Method of Increasing the Future Liver Remnant Volume in the Surgical Treatment of Colorectal Metastases. Arch Surg. 20 Oct 2008;143(10):978.

154. Isfordink CJ, Samim M, Braat MNGJA, Almalki AM, Hagendoorn J, Borel Rinkes IHM, et al. Portal vein ligation versus portal vein embolization for induction of hypertrophy of the future liver remnant: A systematic review and meta-analysis. Surgical Oncology. sept 2017;26(3):257-67.

155. Van Gulik TM, van den Esschert JW, de Graaf W, van Lienden KP, Busch ORC, Heger M, et al. Controversies in the Use of Portal Vein Embolization. Dig Surg. 2008;25(6):436-44.

156. Farges O, Denys A. Portal embolization before hepatectomy. Techniques, indications and results. Annales de Chirurgie. Nov 2001;126(9):836-44.

157. Nagino M, Ando M, Kamiya J, Uesaka K, Sano T, Nimura Y. Liver regeneration after major hepatectomy for biliary cancer: Liver regeneration after major hepatectomy. Br J Surg. August 2001;88(8):1084-91.

158. Corrêa D. Kinetics of Liver Volume Changes in the First Year After Portal Vein Embolization. Arch Surg. Apr 1, 2010;145(4):351.

159. Moris D, Tsilimigras DI, Machairas N, Merath K, Cerullo M, Hasemaki N, et al. Laparoscopic synchronous resection of colorectal cancer and liver metastases: A systematic review. J Surg Oncol. Jan 2019;119(1):30-9.

160. Lin Q, Ye Q, Zhu D, Wei Y, Ren L, Zheng P, et al. Comparison of minimally invasive and open colorectal resections for patients undergoing simultaneous R0 resection for liver metastases: a propensity score analysis. Int J Colorectal Dis. March 2015;30(3):385-95.

161. Gorgun E, Yazici P, Onder A, Benlice C, Yigitbas H, Kahramangil B, et al. Laparoscopic versus open 1-stage resection of synchronous liver metastases and primary colorectal cancer. Gland Surg. August 2017;6(4):324-9.

162. Takasu C, Shimada M, Sato H, Miyatani T, Imura S, Morine Y, et al. Benefits of simultaneous laparoscopic resection of primary colorectal cancer and liver metastases: Simultaneous laparoscopic resection of LM. Asian J Endosc Surg. jan 2014;7(1):31-7.

163. Hu M, Ou-yang C, Liu R. Outcomes of Open Versus Laparoscopic Procedure for Synchronous Radical Resection of Liver Metastatic Colorectal Cancer: A Comparative Study. Surg Laparosc Endosc Percutan Tech. 2012;22(4):6.

164. Chen K-Y, Xiang G-A, Wang H-N, Xiao F-L. Simultaneous laparoscopic excision for rectal carcinoma and synchronous hepatic metastasis. Chin Med J. Oct 2011;124(19):2990-2.

165. Ivanecz A, Krebs B, Stozer A, Jagric T, Plahuta I, Potrc S. Simultaneous pure laparoscopic resection of primary colorectal cancer and synchronous liver metastases: a single institution experience with propensity score matching analysis. Radiology and Oncology. Nov 1, 2017;52(1):42-53.

166. Xu X, Guo Y, Chen G, Li C, Wang H, Dong G. Laparoscopic resections of colorectal cancer and synchronous liver metastases: a case controlled study. Minimally Invasive Therapy & Allied Technologies. 4 Jul 2018;27(4):209-16.

167. Gérard J-P, André T, Bibeau F, Conroy T, Legoux J-L, Portier G, et al. Rectal cancer: French Intergroup clinical practice guidelines for diagnosis, treatments and follow-up (SNFGE, FFCD, GERCOR, UNICANCER, SFCD, SFED, SFRO). Digestive and Liver Disease. Apr 2017;49(4):359-67.

168. Clavien PA, Sanabria JR, Strasberg SM. Proposed classification of complications of surgery with examples of utility in cholecystectomy. Surgery. May 1992;111(5):518-26.

169. JL C, H J. Prospective evaluation of perioperative adverse events in laparoscopic surgery. e-memoires de l'Académie nationale de chirurgie. 2015;(Vol.14, fasc.4):50-5.

170 Clavien P-A, Vetter D, Staiger RD, Slankamenac K, Mehra T, Graf R, et al. The Comprehensive Complication Index (CCI®): Added Value and Clinical Perspectives 3 Years "Down the Line". Annals of Surgery. June 2017;265(6):1045-50.

171. Kim SH, Lim S-B, Ha YH, Han S-S, Park SJ, Choi HS, et al. Laparoscopic-Assisted Combined Colon and Liver Resection for Primary Colorectal Cancer with Synchronous Liver Metastases: Initial Experience. World J Surg. Dec 2008;32(12):2701-6.

172. M.-F. YE, G.-G. XU. Safety and efficacy evaluation of laparoscopy in colorectal cancer with liver metastasis. :6.

173. Aljiffry M, Alrajraji M, Hassanain M, Al-Sabah S. Laparoscopic-assisted one-stage resection of rectal cancer with synchronous liver metastasis utilizing a pfannenstiel incision. Saudi J Gastroenterol. 2014;20(5):315.

174. Ratti F, Catena M, Di Palo S, Staudacher C, Aldrighetti L. Impact of totally laparoscopic combined management of colorectal cancer with synchronous hepatic metastases on severity of complications: a propensity-score-based analysis. Surg Endosc. nov 2016;30(11):4934-45.

175. Uk JK, Cheol KH, Beom CY, David KCH, Hyeon YS, Seok HJ, et al. Outcomes of Simultaneous Laparoscopic Colorectal and Hepatic Resection for Patients with Colorectal Cancers: A Comparative Study. :7.

176. Amajoyi R, Lee Y, Recio PJ, Kondylis PD. Neoadjuvant therapy for rectal cancer decreases the number of lymph nodes harvested in operative specimens. The American Journal of Surgery. March 2013;205(3):289-92.

177. Chang KH, Kelly NP, Duff GP, Condon ET, Waldron D, Coffey JC. Neoadjuvant therapy does not affect lymph node ratio in rectal cancer. The Surgeon. oct 2016;14(5):270-3.

178. Sawayama H, Hayashi N, Honda S, Baba Y, Toyama E, Watanabe M, et al. Treatment results of FOLFOX chemotherapy before surgery for lymph node metastasis of advanced colorectal cancer with synchronous liver metastasis: the status of LN metastasis and vessel invasions at the primary site in patients who responded to FOLFOX. Int J Clin Oncol. Feb 2010;15(1):70-6.

179. Karoui M, Koubaa W, Delbaldo C, Charachon A, Laurent A, Piedbois P, et al. Chemotherapy Has Also an Effect on Primary Tumor in Colon Carcinoma. Ann Surg Oncol. Dec 2008;15(12):3440-6.

180. Ramia-Angel JM. Complete clinical response of liver metastasis after chemotherapy: To resect or not? WJGO. 2011;3(7):107.

181. Lokuhetty D, World Health Organization, International Agency for Research on Cancer. WHO classification of tumours. 2019.

182. Chen Y-W, Huang M-T, Chang T-C. Long term outcomes of simultaneous laparoscopic versus open resection for colorectal cancer with synchronous liver metastases. Asian Journal of Surgery. jan 2019;42(1):217-23.

183. Xu J-M. Robot-assisted one-stage resection of rectal cancer with liver and lung metastases. WJG. 2015;21(9):2848.

184. Karoui M, Scatton O. The "Short-Cut" Laparoscopic Reverse Approach: A Novel Strategy for Synchronous Colorectal Cancer and Liver Metastases Requiring Major or Complex Procedures? World J Surg. August 2019;43(8):2086-9.

# XIV. Appendices :

## *Appendix 1: Patient information sheet.*

### FICHE TECHNIQUE

Rang :............ N° Dossier :..................
Nom :................................... Prénom :.................................................
Nom de jeune fille :......................................................
Sexe : Masculin □ Féminin □
Situation familiale :......................................................
Date de naissance :............................................... Age :.....................
Adresse :...................................................................................................
Numéro de téléphone :..........................................
Profession :.............................................
Date de consultation :...............................................................
Date d'entrée :......................................................................
Date d'intervention :.............................................................
Date de sortie :......................................................................
Mode de sortie :.....................................................................

---

Diagnostic :..................................................................................
..................................................................................................
Geste opératoire :..........................................................................
..................................................................................................

---

**Antécédents :**
Personnels...........................................
Facteurs de risque...................................
Médicaments.........................................
ASA....................................I. II. III. IV
Notion de cancer familiale.......oui □ non □
PRC...................................oui □ non □
HNPCC...............................oui □ non □

**Examen général :**
Poids :........Kg Taille :.......cm
BMI :..............Kg/m²
Taux d'amaigrissement................%
Score OMS...............0 □ I □ II □ III □
Indice de Karnofsky....................%

---

**Clinique :**
Début des troubles :.............................
Syndrome rectal..............................oui □ non □
Epreintes.................................oui □ non □
Ténesme..................................oui □ non □
Rectorragie........................ ..... oui □ non □
Diarrhée................................. .oui □ non □
Constipation.......................... .. oui □ non □
Proctalgies.............................. oui □ non □
Mélénas................................. oui □ non □
Syndrome occlusif...........................oui □ non □
Amaigrissement........................... oui □ non □
Anémie...................................... oui □ non □
Autres :.......................................................

**Examen digestif :**
HPMG...............................oui □ non □
Masse palpable.....................oui □ non □
SPMG.................................oui □ non □
Cicatrice de chirurgie Abd....oui □ non □
ADP inguinale....................oui □ non □
Autres..............................................

---

**Examen Proctologique**
Examen de la marge anale
Cloison pubo-anale..........Souple □ Infiltrée □
Cloison ano-coccygienne...Souple □ Infiltrée □
Fistule Périnéale..............................oui □ non □
Toucher Rectal
Pole Inferieure de la tumeur................cm/MA
Circonférence...................¼ □ ½ □ ¾ □ 4/4 □
Situation....Ant □ Post □ Lat Dt □ Lat Gche □
Fixité.......................................oui □ non □
Pole Supérieure perçu.................oui □ non □

Taille Tumorale......................cm
Cloison rectovaginale...Souple □ Infiltrée □
Etat du sphincter anal :
Sans contraction
bonne qualité □ mauvaise qualité □
Avec contraction
bonne qualité □ mauvaise qualité □
Toucher vaginal
Cloison rectovaginale.......Souple □ infiltrée □
Fistule rectovaginale.............oui □ non □

**Rectosigmoidoscopie**
Siège
Marge Anale.......................................cm
Ligne Pectinée....................................cm
Macroscopie.......................................
Circonférence.................¼ □ ½ □ ¾ □ 4/4 □
Sténosant...............................oui □ non □
Taille...............................................cm
Lésions associées.......................................
Biopsie...................................................
Colonoscopie...............................................
.................................................................
**Colo-scanner**
Normal □ polype □ cancer synchrone □
**Echo-endoscopie**
T1 □ T2 □ T3 □ T4 □ N- □ N+ □

**IRM**
T1 □ T2 □ T3 □ T4 □ N- □ N+ □
Graisse périrectale saine...............oui □ non □
T1a □ T1b □ T1c □ T1d □
Epaississement...............................mm
Marge distale sphincter......................mm
Marge circonférentielle......................mm
Distance marge anale.....................mm
Sphincter interne infiltré .............oui □ non □
EIS infiltré..................................oui □ non □
Sphincter externe infiltré..............oui □ non □
Muscles releveurs infiltrés........oui □ non □
Paroi pelvienne infiltrée...............oui □ non □
Organes génitaux internes infiltrés...oui □ non □

**TDM - TAP**
Ganglions ...........................oui □ non □
Siège...............................................
Foie :
Nombre ............................................
Bilobaire ............................oui □ non □
Siège :
Segments..........................................
Sous capsulaire...................................
Profonde..........................................
Taille ...............................................
Voir Schéma de cartographie des lésions

**Classification préthérapeutique cTNM :**
.....................................................

**Biologie**
Groupe Sanguin...........................................
Hb........................................................g/dl
GB............................................ Elets/mm³
Plaq............................................ Elets/mm³
Lymphocytes..................................Elets/mm³
Albumine...................................................g/l
Bilan hépatique ALAT........ASAT........
γGT.........PA........TP......%
Bilan rénal Urée......mg/l Créat.........g/l
Glycémie...................................................g/l
Na +.................../K+............................
ACE.................. CA19-9........................

**Opérabilité :**

ASA.....................................I. II. III. IV.
Score OMS..............0 □ I □ II □ III □
Indice de Karnofsky....................%
Fonction cardiaque ...............FE.........%
Fonction respiratoire............................
Consultation de pré anesthésie faite le .................
Par le Dr......................................................

**Bilan nutritionnel :**

Poids :........Kg Taille :.......cm
BMI :..............Kg/m²
Taux d'amaigrissement................%
Lymphocytes...................................Elets/mm³
Albumine...................................................g/l

**Préparation à la chirurgie :**

Transfusion sanguine........................oui □ non □
Alimentation parentérale.....................oui □ non □
Régime alimentaire spécifique............oui □ non □
Traitement médical..........................oui □ non □

**Stratégie thérapeutique :**

.................................................................
.................................................................
.................................................................

RT néo adjuvante :

Protocole :...................................................
Date de début :...............................................
Date de fin :...................................................
Par Dr.........................................................
Toxicité.......................................................
.................................................................
Réévaluation.................................................
.................................................................
.................................................................

CT péri opératoire :

Protocole :...................................................
Date de début :...............................................
Date de fin :...................................................
Par Dr.........................................................
Toxicité.......................................................
.................................................................
Réévaluation.................................................
.................................................................
.................................................................

**Intervention :**

Date d'intervention :…………………………………..
Salle opératoire :…………………………………….
Chirurgien :…………………………………………..
Aides opératoires :……………………………………
Médecin réanimateur :………………………………
Instrumentiste :……………………………………..

Voie d'abord :
Nombre de trocarts……………………………….
Dispo des trocarts……………………………………….
………………………………………………………………
Incisions…………………………………………………
………………………………………………………………
Longueur des cicatrices……………………………..
………………………………………………………………
Voir schéma en annexe

Exploration :……………………………………………
……………………………………………………………..
……………………………………………………………..

Geste opératoire :……………………………………..
……………………………………………………………..
Colon/rectum…………………………………………
……………………………………………………………..
Foie…………………………………………………………
……………………………………………………………..

Gestes associés…………………………………………
……………………………………………………………..

Type de drainage……………………………………..
……………………………………………………………

Transfusion sanguine per -op ……….. oui □ non □
…………………………………………………………

Incidents per-op :………………………………………
………………………………………………………………
………………………………………………………………

Temps opératoire global ………………………..mn
Temps opératoire (primitif)……………………..mn
Temps opératoire (Méta)………………………..mn

Pertes Sanguines……………………………….cc

Analgésie per opératoire (Marcaïne)…. oui □ non □

Schéma d'analgésie per et post opératoire…………
……………………………………………………………
……………………………………………………………
……………………………………………………………

Séjour en réanimation ……………….. oui □ non □
Durée…………………………………….jours

Alimentation parentérale ……………. oui □ non □

**Morbidité postopératoire :**

**Médicale…………………………oui □ non □**

Σd respiratoire □ Σd cardiovasculaire □
Σd métabolique □ Σd infectieux □

**Chirurgicale**

Hémorragie……………..……………oui □ non □
PPO……………………………………oui □ non □
Nécrose colique……...……………..oui □ non □
Fistules anastomotiques…………..oui □ non □
Fistule réctovaginale…...…………oui □ non □
Eviscération………………………...oui □ non □
Suppuration pariétale……………..oui □ non □
Complications stomiales……...…..oui □ non □
Autres :……………………………………………..
…………………………………………………………

Classification de Clavien - Dindo …………………
……………………………………………………………

Délai post opératoire :……………………………..

Signes d'appel :………………………………………
……………………………………………………………

Biologie :………………………………………………
……………………………………………………………
……………………………………………………………

Morphologie :…………………………………………
……………………………………………………………
……………………………………………………………

Traitement :……………………………………………
……………………………………………………………
……………………………………………………………

**Réintervention**
Délai : ……………………………….
Cause :…………………………………………………..
Exploration opératoire :……………………………..
……………………………………………………………..
Bactériologie :…………………………………………..
Geste opératoire :……………………………………..
……………………………………………………………
Evolution :……………………………………………..
……………………………………………………………

**Mortalité post opératoire :**
Cause :…………………………………………………..
Délai :……………………………………………………..

**Anatomie pathologique :**
**Macroscopie**
Pièce fraîche □
Pièce fixée étalée □
Localisation tumorale :
Haut rectum □ Moyen rectum □ Bas rectum □
Colon □
Longueur de la résection……………………cm
Marge Proximale……………………………cm
Marge Distale………………………………cm
Qualité du mésorectum
Complet □ Presque complet □ Incomplet □
Taille tumorale
Hauteur……………………………………….. cm
Longueur……………………………………… cm
Epaisseur………………………………………cm
Circonférence…………………..¼ □ ½ □ ¾ □ 4/4 □
Aspect
Plan □ Bourgeonnant □ Infiltrant □ Mixte □
Séreuse infiltrée…………………………oui □ non □
Perforation………………………………oui □ non □
Polypes…………………………………...oui □ non □
Nombre de ganglions prélevés……………………...
Localisation……………………………………………
Métastase (s) …………………………………………
……………………………………………………………
Autres……………………………………………………

**Examen histologique**
**Adénocarcinome**
ADK bien≠ □ ADK Moy≠ □ ADK In≠ □
Colloïde Muqueux □
Composante colloïde………………………………%
Autres……………………………………………………
**Infiltration pariétale** :
Muqueuse □ s/ muqueuse □ musculeuse □
s/séreuse □ séreuse □
**Grade de régression tumorale**
**Grade I**……………………Régression complète □
**Grade II**
Rares Cellules tumorale dans une fibrose dense □
**Grade III**
Cellules Tumorales développée dans la fibrose □
**Grade IV**
Cellules Tumorales à l'extérieure de la fibrose □
**Grade V**…………………….. Absence de réponse □
Infiltration du canal anal………………oui □ non □
Infiltration d'un autre organe………… oui □ non □
Marge Distale
Saine □ Infiltrée □
Marge de résection circonférentielle……………mm
Nombre de ganglions prélevés……………………….
Nombre de ganglions métastatiques………………...
N+/N……………………………………………………
Embols Vasculaires………………………oui □ non □
Intramuraux □ Extramuraux □
Infiltration Péri Nerveuse……………..oui □ non □
Autres……………………………………………………
Résidu tumoral…………… R0 □ R1 □ R2 □
Radiothérapie…………………………..oui □ non □
Protocole (Si oui)…………………………………..
Radio chimiothérapie…………………oui □ non □

**Statut p/ ypTNM**
T0 □ T1 □ T2 □ T3 □ T4 □
N1 □ N2 □ Nx □
M0 □ M1 □ Mx □
Statut MSI…………………………………………………
Statut Ki-ras ………………………………………………

Méta hépatique :
Type histologique……………………………………….
……………………………………………………………
Limites de résection……………………………………
……………………………………………………………
TRG………………………………………………………
……………………………………………………………
Résidu tumoral…………… R0 □ R1 □ R2 □

Nom du pathologiste :

**Traitement Adjuvant** ………………….. oui □ non □
Protocole :………………………………………………
Date de début :………………………………………...
Date de fin :……………………………………………
Par Dr……………………………………………………
Toxicité…………………………………………………
……………………………………………………………
Réévaluation……………………………………………
……………………………………………………………
……………………………………………………………

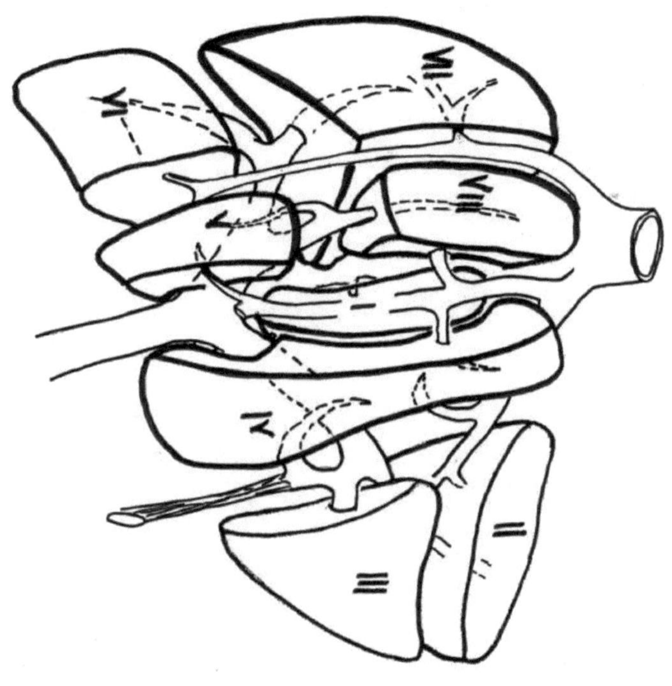


Schematic diagram of liver segmentation, part of the patient information sheet, to record the number, size and location of metastases.

**Fellow-up :**

.............................................................................................................................

...........

.............................................................................................................................

...........

.............................................................................................................................

...........

………………………………………………………………………………………………………
…………

………………………………………………………………………………………………………
…………

………………………………………………………………………………………………………
…………

………………………………………………………………………………………………………
…………

………………………………………………………………………………………………………
…………

***Appendix 2:*** *Chemotherapy protocols.*

## Protocole FOLFOX4 simplifié

**Durée d'une cure : 2 jours ; intervalle entre 2 cures : 2 semaines (J1=J15)**

J1
• **Oxaliplatine ELOXATINE®: 85 mg/m$^2$**
en perfusion IV de 120 min (en Y avec l'acide folinique)
• **Acide folinique : 400 mg/m$^2$ ou Acide L-folinique : 200 mg/m$^2$**
en perfusion IV de 120 min (en Y avec l'oxaliplatine)
• **5-Fluoro-uracile « bolus » : 400 mg/m$^2$**
en perfusion IV de 10 min
• **5-Fluoro-uracile « infusionnel »: 1200 mg/m$^2$**
en infusion IV continue de 22h (infuseur ou pompe)*

J2
• **5-Fluoro-uracile « infusionnel »: 1200 mg/m$^2$**
en infusion IV continue de 24h (infuseur ou pompe)*

* en pratique, mise en place à J1 d'une infusion intraveineuse continue de 46 heures de 2400 mg/m$^2$ de 5-fluoro-uracile

## Protocole XELOX

**Durée d'une cure : 2 semaines; intervalle entre 2 cures : 3 semaines (J1=J22)**

J1
• **Oxaliplatine ELOXATINE® : 130 mg/m$^2$**
en perfusion IV de 2 heures

J2 à J15 inclus :
• **Capécitabine XELODA® : 1000 mg/m$^2$ matin et soir (soit 2000 mg/m$^2$/j)***
par voie orale (prise des comprimés avec un peu d'eau dans les 30 minutes suivant la fin du petit déjeuner et du dîner)

**J16 à J21 inclus : Pas de traitement**

**Attention* : posologie inférieure à celle de la capécitabine prescrite en monothérapie*

## ***Appendix 3:*** *AGER protocol*



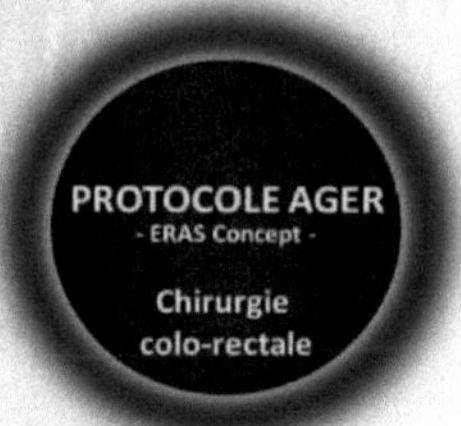


**AGER**
**Algerian Group of Enhanced Recovery**

***Objectifs du protocole AGER:***

- Réduire la morbidité
- Réduire le séjour hospitalier
- Réduire les couts d'hospitalisation

### 1. Phase Préopératoire

a) **Information du patient en pré opératoire**: lors des 2 consultations chirurgie et anesthésie.

b) **Modalités du jeûne :**
- Liquides sucrés (eau sucrée, tisanes sucrées....) jusqu'à **2 h** avant l'induction
- Apport solides (biscottes, biscuits..), jusqu'à **6 h** avant l'induction
- Diabétique (type 2) bien équilibré, idem
- Diabétique (type 1) avec neuropathie, jeûne aux solides à partir de minuit et liquides autorisés jusqu'à **3 h** avant induction

* Tabac : sevrage avant la chirurgie

c) **Préparation colique :**
- Chirurgie du côlon : non
- Chirurgie du rectum
  - Amputation abdominopérinéale : non
  - Rétablissement de continuité : oui
    - * Préparation mécanique et lavement rectal
    - * Si tumeur sténosante lavement rectal seul

d) **Prémédication :** Aucune prémédication

e) **Thromboprophylaxie : HBPM** minimum **12 h** avant ou **6 - 8 h** après

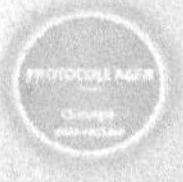

## 2. Phase Peropératoire

a) **Antibioprophylaxie : 30 à 60 mn** avant incision:

- *Protocole 1:* **Cefotaxime** en **IV** en dose unique + **Imidazolé 1g** en **perfusion** et en dose unique **Ou**

- *Protocole 2:* **Aminopénicilline** + inhibiteurs des **bétalactamases** (**Augmentin***) : **2 g** en **IV lente** en dose unique. Si durée **> 2 h,** réinjecter **1g** **Ou**

- *Protocole 3:* **Ertapénème, 1g / J** si **FDR de E-BLSE**. (voir annexe) **Ou**

Si **allergie** aux bétalactamines :

- *Protocole 4:* **Imidazolé** 1g + **Gentamycine 5 mg / kg / j** en perfusion et en dose unique.

b) **Thromboprophylaxie :** Bas de contention

c) **Monitorage de la volémie :** restriction monitorée des apports liquidiens

d) **Techniques anesthésiques et monitorage de la curarisation :**
- Privilégier les narcotiques à durée d'action courte : **Propofol**, **Sevoflurane**
- Eviter N2O si possible
- Privilégier **Rocuronium** et **Vecuronium**.

Monitorage de la curarisation (NMT) par le recours au Train de quatre (TOF) avec comme objectif du bloc neuromusculaire (BNM) : profond (laparotomie) ou très profond (laparoscopie).
- Si laparotomie : réponse **0** à **1/4**, réinjection dès **2/4**
- Si laparoscopie: réponse **0/4**, réinjection dès **1/4**

e) **Lutte contre l'hypothermie :** (objectif T° **> 36° C**):
- Réchauffement corporel (couverture chauffante à air chaud, matelas chauffant...)
- Réchauffement des solutés à perfuser ou d'irrigation péritonéale.

f) **Abord chirurgical:**
- Laparotomie
- Laparoscopie à privilégier

g) **Drainage :**
- Chirurgie colique : non sauf cas particulier
- Chirurgie rectale : oui, aspiratif **48** à **72 h**

h) **Nausées/vomissements :** Prévention multimodale
- **Dexaméthasone 8 mg** à l'induction
- **Ondansetron 4 mg** en fin d'intervention si score d'Apfel **≥ 2** (voir annexe)

i) **Analgésie :**
- **Paracétamol**, **1g** perfusion, **45 min** avant fin chirurgie
- **Kétamine** en perfusion si FDR d'hyperalgésie centrale (douleur, opioïdes et anxiété – dépression préopératoires) : **0,5mg / kg** en induction puis **0,25mg / kg** si chirurgie prévue **> 2h**, arrêt **30 mn** avant réveil. (voir annexe)

## 3. Phase Postopératoire

a) **Antagonisation de la curarisation selon le monitorage NMT :**

- TOF **> 75% :** extubation **sans** décurarisation pharmacologique
- TOF **25 - 75%,** ou **3 - 4** réponses : **Sugammadex, 2mg/Kg**
- TOF **1 - 2** réponses : **Sugammadex 4mg/Kg**

b) **Analgésie multimodale :**

- Péridurale dorsale : **Ropivacaine** ou **Bupivacaine** + **Sufentanil** soit à la SAP ou via une pompe elastomérique, durée **2 à 3 jours**

NB : Pose en préopératoire (ou en postopératoire si nécessaire)

- Si pas de péridurale : **Xylocaine IV 1.5mg / kg / h IV continue** ou **TAP** bloc bilatéral, single shoot : **Ropivacaine** ou **Bupivacaine.**

Quelque soit la technique, associer **Paracétamol 1g X 4 / J** relais voie orale à partir de **J2 - J3**

> - Si insuffisant : **AINS, Acupan 20mg 4 X / J** ou **Tramadol**
> - Si insuffisant : **Morphine,** titration **IV** puis administration idéalement **PCA** (électronique ou mécanique), sinon **S/C** chaque **6H**.

c) **Ablation de la sonde nasogastrique en fin d'intervention**

d) **Ablation de la sonde urinaire :**

- Dans les **24 H**
- **> 24H** si maintien de la péridurale, chirurgie du cancer du rectum, dissection antérieure difficile, brèche vésicale ou urétrale, parésie vésicale.

e) **Alimentation orale précoce :**

- **J0 :** Boissons selon la tolérance
- **J1 :** Eau, tisanes sucrées + chewing gum*, bonbons à sucer, compote
- **J2 :** Eau, tisanes sucrées + bouillon de légumes + fromage en portions
- **J3 :** Eau, tisanes, thé, café, fromage, bouillon matin, purée le soir, crème-dessert

f) **Mobilisation précoce / kinésithérapie**

- **J1 :** Mise au fauteuil
- **J2 :** Quelques pas dans la chambre
- **J3 :** Déambulation dans le couloir

g) **Thromboprophylaxie : HBPM 6 h à 8 h** post opératoire et poursuivre pendant un mois si chirurgie carcinologique ou inflammatoire (MICI)

**Sortie à partir de J5 sauf complication**

***Appendix 4:*** *Apfel score.*

| | Oui | Non | Score d'Apfel | Risques de NVPO |
|---|---|---|---|---|
| Sexe féminin | 1 | 0 | 0 | < 10 % |
| Tabagisme | 0 | 1 | 1 | 21 % |
| Antécédents de NVPO et/ ou de mal des transports | 1 | 0 | 2 | 39 % |
| Morphine post-opératoire | 1 | 0 | 3 | 61 % |
| Score d'Apfel | 0 à 4 | | 4 | 79 % |

***Appendix 5:*** *Modified Aldrete score.*

| SCORE D'ALDRETE | | | | | |
|---|---|---|---|---|---|
| | **Activité** | **Respiration** | **Circulation** | **Conscience** | **Saturation pulsée en oxygène** |
| 2 pts | Bouge les 4 membres à la demande | Respire profondément et peut tousser sans difficulté | PA ± 20 % de la valeur pré-anesthésique | Complètement réveillé | $SpO_2$ > 92% à l'air |
| 1 pt | Bouge 2 membres | Dyspnéique, respiration superficielle ou limitée | PA ± 20-50 % de la valeur pré-anesthésique | Réveillable à l'appel | Apport d'$O_2$ nécessaire pour maintenir une $SpO_2$ > 90% |
| 0 pt | Ne bouge aucun membre | Apnéique | PA ± 50 % de la valeur pré-anesthésique | Aucun réveil à l'appel | SpO2 < 92% malgé supplémentation en $O_2$ |

***Appendix 6:*** *WHO performance status.*

## PERFORMANCE STATUS DE L'OMS

| Activité | Score |
|---|---|
| | |
| **Capable d'une activité identique à celle précédant la maladie** | 0 |
| **Activité physique diminuée, mais ambulatoire et capable de mener un travail** | 1 |
| **Ambulatoire et capable de prendre soin de soi-même. Incapable de travailler et alité moins de 50% du temps** | 2 |
| **Capable seulement de quelques activités. Alité ou en chaise plus de 50% du temps** | 3 |
| **Incapable de prendre soin de soi-même. Alité ou en chaise en permanence** | 4 |

***Appendix 7:*** *Classification of the severity of anastomotic fistulas after anterior resection.*

| | | |
|---|---|---|
| Definition | Defect of the intestinal wall integrity at the colorectal or colo-anal anastomotic site (including suture and staple lines of neorectal reservoirs) leading to a communication between the intra- and extraluminal compartments. A pelvic abscess close to the anastomosis is also considered as anastomotic leakage. | |
| Grade | A | Anastomotic leakage requiring no active therapeutic intervention |
| | B | Anastomotic leakage requiring active therapeutic intervention but manageable without re-laparotomy |
| | C | Anastomotic leakage requiring re-laparotomy |

***Appendix 8:*** *The complete complication index and the CCI®Calculator.*

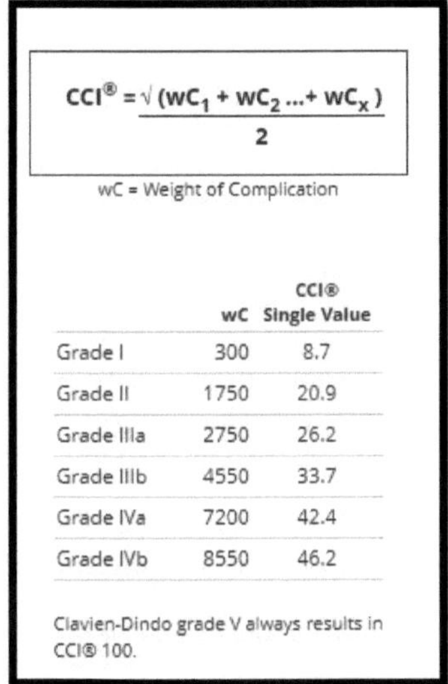

$$CCI^{®} = \frac{\sqrt{(wC_1 + wC_2 ... + wC_x)}}{2}$$

wC = Weight of Complication

| | wC | CCI® Single Value |
|---|---|---|
| Grade I | 300 | 8.7 |
| Grade II | 1750 | 20.9 |
| Grade IIIa | 2750 | 26.2 |
| Grade IIIb | 4550 | 33.7 |
| Grade IVa | 7200 | 42.4 |
| Grade IVb | 8550 | 46.2 |

Clavien-Dindo grade V always results in CCI® 100.

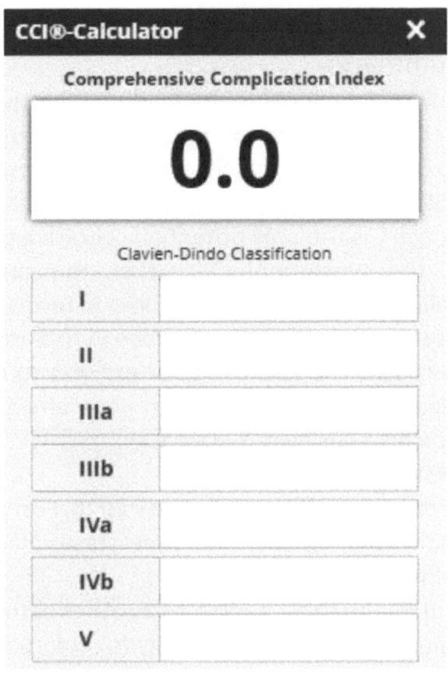

# XV. Abstracts :

Summary:
Colorectal cancer is the leading digestive cancer in Algeria. The liver is the most frequent site of colorectal cancer metastases. During the course of the disease, 40 to 60% of patients will develop liver metastases, which are synchronous in 10 to 25% of cases.
Surgery is the only potentially curative treatment.
In the synchronous situation, the simultaneous surgical approach has been validated, but poses a problem in terms of approach.
Laparoscopy may have a place in this approach.
Purpose: The aim of our study was to evaluate the feasibility and safety of the laparoscopic approach in combined surgery for colorectal cancer with synchronous liver metastases.
Materials and methods:
From August 2016 to January 2020, Forty patients with colorectal adenocarcinoma with synchronous liver metastases had been approached laparoscopically for combined surgery.
During the same period, forty other patients with colorectal adenocarcinoma were approached laparoscopically for colorectal excision surgery alone.
Perioperative results of combined laparoscopic surgery as well as oncological outcomes had been evaluated.
The immediate results of the two study arms were compared.
Results: In combined surgery, 4 patients had a totally laparoscopic approach, 24 patients a hybrid approach and 9 patients down-staging surgery. We converted 3 patients (conversion rate 7.5%).
The overall morbidity rate in the combined surgery arm was 27.5%, while the mortality rate was zero.
Colorectal surgery was R0 in 95% of cases, liver surgery was R0 in 92.8% of cases.
Nine patients had a recurrence during the follow-up period.
All patients were alive at the point date.
Mean recurrence-free survival was 28.91 months, median recurrence-free survival 27 months.
Comparison between the two study arms found no difference in morbidity rates, fistula rates, conversion rates and postoperative stay, but combined surgery was significantly longer.

Conclusion: The results of our study support the feasibility of laparoscopy in the management of colorectal cancer with synchronous liver metastases in selected patients.
Key words: Colorectal cancer - Synchronous liver metastases - Laparoscopy - Simultaneous surgery.

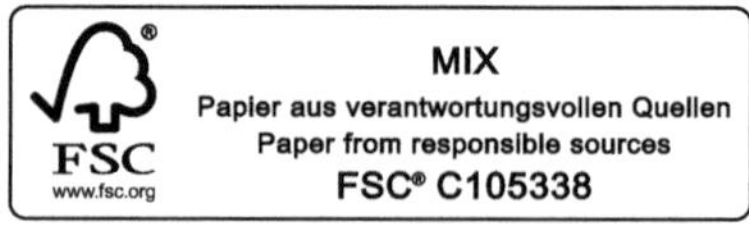


Printed by Books on Demand GmbH, Norderstedt / Germany